Evidence-Based Occlusal Management for Temporomandibular Disorders

Authored By

Kengo Torii

General Dentistry of the Infirmary
School of Life Dentistry
Nippon Dental University
Tokyo
Japan

CONTENTS

FOREWORD

Professor Torii has put together a well-balanced treatise on the concept of an occlusal basis as a risk indicator while still keeping the evidence for a bio psychosocial intervention in patients with T.M. disorders.

I am particularly impressed that the concepts put forward by Professor Torii have been supported by the literature he has reviewed.

This treatise is a must for students and practitioners who wish to successfully treat patients with Temporomandibular Disorders by combining dental and medical concepts into an effective management philosophy.

Noshir R. Mehta
Tufts University School of Dental Medicine
Boston
Massachusetts
USA

PREFACE

Although the role of occlusion in the manifestation of the signs and symptoms associated with temporomandibular disorders (TMDs) remains controversial, occlusal adjustment or occlusal reconstruction therapies have been undertaken for the treatment of TMDs. However, a joint conference of the National Institute of Health (NIH) and National Institute of Dental Research (NIDR) held in May 1996 in the USA concluded that occlusion and TMDs were not related, and this decision has definitely affected clinicians and researchers. Since then, many well-known TMD clinicians and researchers have not alluded to any relation between occlusion and TMDs, and treatment for TMD has shifted to more conservative modalities. However, we have never been convinced that all the evidence completely rules out a possible relation between occlusion and TMDs. Recently, the relation of a discrepancy between the habitual occlusal position (HOP) and the bite plate-induced occlusal position (BPOP) to TMD has been reported. Thus, the possible effect of the occlusal equilibration of the BPOP on TMD signs and symptoms has also been inferred. We previously reported the transient effects of conservative therapies on TMD and highlighted the need for occlusal equilibration of the BPOP.

Here, our description, together with the colored pictorial representation, covers the following points:

1. When do the signs or symptoms of TMD appear?

2. Should the signs or symptoms be left untreated?

3. When should treatment start?

4. How should the occlusal discrepancy be examined?

5. How should occlusion at the BPOP be equilibrated?

The aim of this study is to provide a better understanding of the importance of occlusal equilibration in the masticatory muscles-guided position for TMD. We will demonstrate how to equilibrate the patient's occlusion according to the magnitude of the occlusal discrepancy and how to use an articulator for the occlusal equilibration. Although TMD is not a fatal disease, the quality of the patient's life is affected because of the associated headaches, aural symptoms, masticatory dysfunction and posture. Since the expert's panel of the NIDR was met in 1996, an ugly conflict has arisen and persists between the occlusal treatment school and the conservative treatment school. Conservative treatments are reversible, therefore, the treatments are thought to benefit TMD patients at present. However, we have reported that the effects of these conservative treatments for TMD are transitory and recurrence inevitably occurs. We have obtained a good outcome using causal treatment (occlusal equilibration in the BPOP) based on the evidence of a relation between occlusal discrepancy and TMD. Therefore, our clinical data should be shared with many clinicians throughout the world.

ACKNOWLEDGEMENTS

Declared none.

CONFLICT OF INTEREST

The author confirms that this ebook content has no conflict of interest.

Kengo Torii

General Dentistry of the Infirmary
School of Life Dentistry
Nippon Dental University
Tokyo
Japan
E-mail: wbs89508@mail.wbs.ne.jp

Evidence-Based Occlusal Management for Temporomandibular Disorders

Evidence-Based Occlusal Management for Temporomandibular Disorders

2

CHAPTER 1

Prevalence of Temporomandibular Disorders

Abstract: It has been estimated that the prevalence of temporomandibular disorders is in 20-30% of population, but the need for treatment is in less than 5%. However, early treatment is needed for individuals with limitation of opening mouth or pain during mandibular function.

Keywords: Temporomandibular disorders, temoromandibular joint, epidemiological study, cross-sectional study, TMJ clicking, parafunction, lip biting, tongue biting, nail biting, facial pain, locking, bruxism, headache.

1. INTRODUCTION

Epidemiological studies have mainly been conducted in Scandinavian countries since 1970's to analyze the etiologies of temporomandibular disorders (TMDs), to prevent and control TMD and to supply the information on the assessment of needs and potential demands for the treatment of TMDs. Initially, cross-sectional studies were performed, followed by longitudinal studies to investigate the changes of symptoms of TMDs in the course of time.

2. CROSS-SECTIONAL STUDIES

Agerberg and Carlsson investigated individuals of 1,106, aged 15-74 years, and residing in the Swedish city of Umeå by questionnaire regarding the frequency of functional disorders of the masticatory apparatus and certain associated factors (Agerberg G & Carlsson GE, 1972). They reported that facial pain and headache were reported by 24% of the participants, pain on opening mouth was noted in 12%, equally often in males as in females, the limitation of the mandibular movement was reported by 7%, and clicking and crepitation of the temporomandibular joints (TMJ) were reported by 39% individuals. In addition, they reported that pain on movement of the mandible was more common among younger individuals, while other symptoms of dysfunction were relatively equally common in all age groups. They also investigated oral parafunction, such as grinding and clenching of the teeth, biting of the cheek, lip and tongue, and nail biting as the symptoms of TMD. It was concluded that in view of the high frequency of these disorders, the practicing dentist should focus more on the diagnosis and treatment of simple cases of functional disorders of the masticatory apparatus. Helkimo performed a series of studies on the function and dysfunction of the masticatory system. In two populations of Lapps in the north of Finland, 15% reported facial pain, 29. 5% tiredness of the jaw, and 43% were aware of the symptoms related to the movements of the jaw (35% reported TMJ sounds, 9% pain on movement, 8% impaired range of movement, 10% locking and/or luxation) (Helkimo M, 1974). He developed the subjective and clinical indices for dysfunction and occlusal state (Helkimo M, 1974). Hansson and Nilner examined 1069 persons working in a ship-building yard in the south Sweden regarding symptoms of TMDs, and reported that one-fifth of the individuals reported frequent headache and one-fourth of the individuals reported TMJ sounds (Hansson T & Nilner M, 1975). They also reported that clicking of the TMJ was the most common symptom (65%), followed by tenderness of the masticatory musculature to palpation (37%) and tenderness of the TMJ (10%). They estimated that some 25-30% of the individuals examined were in need of treatment. Egermark-Eriksson *et al.* examined 7-, 11-, and 15-year-old Swedish children regarding subjective symptoms and clinical signs of TMDs, and reported that the subjective symptoms (mostly occasional) were reported by 16-25%, with the frequency increasing with age. The prevalence of clinical signs of TMDs also increased with age from 30% in the youngest to 60% in the oldest age group. The most common occurrences of signs were TMJ sounds and tenderness of the masticatory muscles to palpation. In addition, they reported that there was a positive correlation between subjective symptoms and clinical signs of TMDs, as well as between bruxism and clinical signs of TMDs (Egermark-Eriksson I *et al.*, 1981). Nilner and Lassing also reported in 1981 that in 7-14 year old Swedish children (440), the interview revealed 36% with TMD symptoms, 15% with recurrent headaches and 13% reported clicking sounds of TMJs, and 77% of the children reported oral parafunctions (grinding, clenching, lip- and cheek-biting, nail-biting or thumb-sucking) (Nilner M & Lissing S, 1981). In addition, Nilner reported in the same year that in 15-18 year old Swedish adolescents, 41% claimed TMD symptoms, 16% recurrent headaches and 17% had noticed clicking sounds of TMJs (Nilner M, 1981). Similar data as described above were also reported in other articles (Egermark-Eriksson I, 1982; Könönen M, *et al.*, 1987). On the other hand, Heft reported the prevalence of TMJ signs and symptoms in

Caucasian volunteers of U.S.A. He reported that no differences were observed between the old (at least 56 years) and young (less than 56 years) subjects for two or more objective clinical indices; joint noises and deviation of the mandible on opening or closing. A *t*-test of the difference in mm of mouth opening between the old and young groups was significant, showing that the young subjects could open their mouth wider than the old subjects (Heft MW, 1984). Widmalm *et al.* questioned and examined children 4-6 years old, 153 Caucasian and 50 African-American for signs and symptoms of TMDs. They reported that most of the TMD signs and symptoms were mild, and 8% had recurrent (at least 1-2 times per week) TMJ pain, where 5% had recurrent neck pain, in African-American children more often than Caucasian children (Widmalm SE *et al.*, 1995). Thilander *et al.*, divided 4724 children into some groups (deciduous, early mixed, late mixed and permanent dentition) according to the stage of dental development and examined these groups. They reported that one or more clinical signs were recorded in 25% of subjects, most of them being mild in character, and the prevalence increased during the developmental stages (Thilander B *et al.*, 2002). Wahlund examined 864 adolescents from a Public Dental Service clinic (Sweden) and reported that seven percent of the subjects received a pain diagnosis, and the prevalence was higher among girls than boys. Wahlund also compared three treatment methods, and reported that occlusal appliance with a brief information was significantly effective. On the bases of the results of the five studies he elucidated that; (1) Self-administered questions regarding TMD pain and symptoms with a frequency of "once a week or more" are generally more reliable than clinical examination method; (2) Adolescents can be classified into subdiagnoses according to the RDC/TMD with acceptable reliability; (3) Approximately half of the adolescents experiencing pain once a week or more perceived a need for treatment; (4) Psychosocial factors such as increased levels of stress, somatic complaints and emotional problems seem to play a more important role than dental factors in adolescents with TMD pain; and (5) Adolescents with TMD reported significantly more intense experiences to somatic stimuli, whether pleasant or aversive-suggesting that cognitive systems in addition to nociceptive systems are involved (Wahlund K, 2003). Köhler *et al.* concluded from their cross-sectional study that the prevalence of more severe TMD symptoms and signs in children and adolescents was generally low and did not change significantly during the 20-year period. A point that should be emphasized is the need to develop reliable examination methods suitable for children at different levels of cognitive maturity. Further research, including longitudinal epidemiological studies covering the whole span of childhood, is recommended in order to obtain a more comprehensive view of both the natural course of TMD and the factors associated with or predisposing to it, as well as facilitate appropriate treatment at an early stage (Köhler AA *et al.*, 2009). Rugh and Solberg described that knowledge is lacking regarding the natural course of most TMDs, therefore, need for the treatment of TMDs remains unclear. They then concluded that (1) Temporomandibular disorders refer to a wide range of musculoskeletal conditions affecting various aspects of the masticatory system. There are serious definitional problems and no classification scheme has been widely accepted; (2) Although 28-86% of the adult population have one or more signs or symptoms, only 5% are in need of treatment and about the same percentages seek care; (3) Due to the diversity of treatment needs for TM conditions, manpower needs will be spread fairly evenly among general dentists and the various specialties; (4) This patient population, although relatively small in contrast to other dental needs, often has serious disabilities; (5) Current dental educational programs are not adequately training students to manage these patients; (6) There is an immediate need to explore new undergraduate educational programs that provide increased familiarity with diagnostic reasoning, radiology, neurology, physical therapy and pharmacology. In brief, there is a need for increased emphasis on physical diagnosis and the ability to see complex diseases in a psychosocial context; (7) There is a need for advanced training programs to provide the skills necessary to treat more complex TM conditions. Approximately 3-5% of the graduating dentists should undergo this training; and (8) and To meet the needs of patients with TM disorders and to reverse distributing trends in dental continuing education, these new programs are needed immediately. They should receive the highest priority (Rugh JD & Solberg WK, 1985). Lipton *et al.* reported the total number of people with jaw and/or face pain included 7,293 women and 3,481 men with the estimated number of adult population experiencing orofacial pain more than once during the past six months in the United States in 1989. They concluded that an estimated 39 million adults in the U.S. civilian population recently experienced or currently suffer from some type of orofacial pain. As the dentist is often consulted to diagnose or treat these discomforts, the clinician should know all aspects of these conditions, including systemic factors. Since the treatment of patients with pain involves numerous dental and medical specialties, the dental profession must collaborate with clinicians from other disciplines to care for patients, especially those with chronic orofacial pain. The estimated magnitude and distribution of the orofacial pains found in this survey prompt important questions: What is the natural history of these conditions? Which biological, psychological and sociocultural factors may explain the different reported experience of pain in the jaw joint and face for women compared to men? And finally, what were the behavioral and attitudinal responses to pain and the economic cost of the pain to individuals, their employers, insurance carriers and the government? These and other issues should be addressed in future national investigations (Lipton JA *et al.*, 1993). De Kanter *et al.* reported that a total of 21.5% of the Dutch adult population reported dysfunction, but 85% of these perceived no need for treatment, and a figure of 3.1% can be used to summarize the actual level of treatment for TMD in the Dutch adult population (De Kanter RJAM *et al.*, 1992).

3. LONGITUDINAL STUDIES

Magnusson *et al.* conducted a four-year longitudinal study to understand the natural course of signs and subjective symptoms in 119 children (became 11 and 15 from previously 7 and 11 years old). They then reported that the subjective symptoms had increased in frequency in the younger children, while the clinical signs had increased in both groups (Magnusson T *et al.*, 1985). In addition, Magnusson *et al.* performed a five-year longitudinal study in 135 subjects who at the age of 15 years had participated in a cross sectional investigation of TMDs. They reported the only subjective symptom that had changed statistically significantly was TMJ sounds, which had increased between the age of 15 and 20 (Magnusson *et al.*, 1986). De Boever and Van den Berghe reported from their longitudinal study in Flemish children (3 years to 13 years old) that in the most of the children, the TMD symptoms were very mild to moderate and concluded that the treatment need is low and should not be overestimated. In addition, they described that further research should be carried out to define the treatment needs and the high risk group in the child population. Epidemiologic longitudinal studies should help to elucidate the etiology and mechanisms provoking these dysfunctional changes. One can speculate on bruxism, muscle fatigue, occlusion and the psychoemotional tension. However, the present results did not provide any significant answer to the causational problem of TMJ-dysfunctions. This longitudinal study supports the concept that the frequently observed dysfunctional symptoms in children and in adults are not congenital in nature but of a functional origin (De Boever JA & Van den Berghe I, 1987). Wänman reported from a three-year longitudinal study in adolescents (17 years to 19 years old) that TMJ sounds were significantly more often recorded in girls than in boys, and described that a stomatognathic examination should be included in the routine dental check-up to evaluate the frequency, intensity and duration of TMDs, even though the need and demand for treatment may be less significant in adolescents (Wänman A, 1987). Wänman A and Agerberg G described as follows: The number of contacting teeth in the intercuspal position during light pressure was the occlusal factor with the most significant relationships to symptoms of mandibular dysfunction (Wänman A and Agerberg G, 1991). In addition, Wänman reported that the result indicates different courses for CMD in men and women (Wänman A, 1996). Heikinheimo *et al.* reported from their longitudinal study that the symptoms of TMDs did not appear to be consistent and locking of the joint was found to be the most stable symptom. About 50% of those reporting TMJ-clicking, unexplainable ear symptoms or bruxism at the age of 12, had lost this symptom by the age of 15. For pain on mouth-opening, the symptom group at the age of 15 consisted of entirely new individuals. They described that because of their inconsistent nature during the final stages of occlusal development, too much attention should not be paid to single occurrences of TMD symptoms, and symptoms of TMD, recurrent headache, and oral parafunctions should be elicited and recorded at annual dental check-ups of children and adolescents (Heikinheimo K *et al.*, 1989). Könönen and Nyström longitudinally examined 131 Finnish adolescents, and reported that TMJ clicking sounds were most frequent findings and increased with age, however, they showed no predictable pattern, and only a few patients consistently reported clicking sounds or had them recorded (Könönen M & Nyström M, 1993). Magnusson *et al.* reported from their 20 years longitudinal study that progression to severe pain and dysfunction of the masticatory system was rare (Magnusson T *et al.*, 2000). Egermark-Eriksson *et al.* reported that there was a substantial fluctuation of reported symptoms over the 20-year period. Progression to severe pain and dysfunction of the masticatory system was rare. On the other hand, recovery from frequent symptoms to no symptoms was also rare (Egermark-Eriksson I *et al.*, 2001). Rammelsberg *et al.* reported that muscle disorders classified by RDC/TMD are predominantly chronic or fluctuating pain conditions, with a modest probability (31%) of remission (Rammelsberg P *et al.*, 2003). On the other hand, Macfarlane *et al.* performed a cross-sectional population-based survey in the United Kingdom, involving 2504 participants, of whom 646 (26%) reported orofacial pain. Overall, 424 (79%) of these individuals participated in the four-year follow-up, of whom 229 (54%) reported orofacial pain. They summarized that of those persons selected from the community with self-reported orofacial pain, just under half will have symptoms that will resolve after four years. Persons with pain that require medication, other body pain and psychological distress are more likely to be conditions. These findings have important implications for the identification and treatment of patients with orofacial pain (Macfarlane TV *et al.*, 2004). Ahlberg *et al.* described that successful management of TMD necessitates smoking cessation, as tobacco use may both amplify the patient's pain response and provoke bruxism. However, psychosocial factors and perceived stress should not be ignored (Ahlberg J *et al.*, 2004). Nilsson concluded from her study that (1) in 2000, the prevalence of TMD pain among all adolescents aged 12-19 in Östergötland County was 4.2%, being significantly more common among girls than boys, increased significantly with age among both girls and boys, and increased about twice as fast in girls as in boys; (2) One-third of the patients with TMD pain received treatment by dentists; (3) The majority of adolescents with self-reported TMD pain undergo treatment. Almost twice as many girls as boys have a subjective need for TMD treatment; (4) The two self-reported pain questions that constitute the TMD-S variable had very good reliability and high validity; (5) TMD-S can be recommended for use in general screening to detect adolescents with TMD pain; (6) The annual incidence of TMD pain was 2.9%, and the pain pattern fluctuated. Adolescent girls reported higher incidence rate for TMD pain at all ages and for all temporal patterns (Nilsson I, 2007). Marklund and Wönman performed a one-year prospective study on dental students. They concluded that both self-reported bruxism and registered mandibular instability in ICP (intercuspal position) showed association with 1-year period prevalence of myofascial signs and symptoms in the jaw-face region (Marklund S & Wänman A, 2008). Torii performed a five-year longitudinal study on TMJ sounds in Japanese children and adolescents (Torii K, 2011). In his study, no TMDs requiring treatment were observed in the series. TMJ clicking was observed in 30 subjects (48%); however, the clicking was temporary in most of the subjects (26 subjects; 42%), and only 3 subjects (5%) had persistent clicking (continuing until the end of the observation period). The incidences of clicking were not significantly different among the six groups ($x^2 = 4.265$) (Tables **1** and **2**). Clicking was significantly more common among girls (19 subjects) than boys (11subjects; P=0.042) (Table **3**). A significantly lower bite force (17±18 kg) was recorded for the subjects with persistent clicking, compared with that of other subjects (8- and 9-Year-olds; mixed dentition) without persistent clicking (32±17 kg) (Table **4**). Persistent clicking began at the age of 11 or 12 years (permanent dentition) (Table **2**). There was no relation between persistent clicking and the number of decayed, filled or totaly decayed and filled teeth (Table **5**).

Table 1: Contingency table for the number of subjects with and those without TMJ clicking

Group	With Clicking	Without Clicking	Total
G 1	5	4	9
G 2	6	6	12
G 3	3	7	10
G 4	6	7	13
G 5	4	1	5
G 6	8	5	13

$X^2=4.265<X^2(P=0.5)$: not significant.

Table 2: Incidences of TMJ clicking among six age groups

Group	No	1987	1988	1989	1990	1991	1992
	2				□□		
	6		□		□		□
G1	7				□	□	
	10	□	□		□		
	12		□	□□	□□		□
	13				□		
	18	□	□□	□	□□		
G2	21				□		
	23				□		□
	24				□		
	25				□		
	27				□□		
	30		□			□	
G3	31	□		□	■□	□□	□

Table 2: contd…

Group	No.						
	32		□		□		
	33	□					
	34	□					
	37	□					
	38						□
	39			□	□□		
G4	40				□		
	42				□		□
	46		□		□□	□□	□□
	47	□		□			
G5	49				□		
	59		□□	□	□□	□□	■■
	60	□	□		□	□□	■■
G6	65	□	□□	□			
	67						□
	68			□			

G 1: group of subjects aged 5 years old at beginning of observation; G 2: group of subjects aged 6 years old; G 3: group of subjects aged 7 years old; G 4: group of subjects aged 8 years old; G 5: group of subjects aged 9 years old; G 6: group of subjects aged 10 years old. The examinations were performed twice each year except in 1987 and 1989 (only one examination was performed in each of these years). No.: Subject number; □: Clicking; ■: Crepitation.

Table 3: Contingency table for male and female subjects with or without TMJ clickings; Gender with clicking without clicking total

Gender	With Clicking	Without Clicking	Total
Male	11	19	32
Female	19	12	30

P=0.042 (The relationship between girls and clicking was significant when evaluated using the Fisher exact test).

Table 4: Maximum bite force (kg) of subjects with and without persistent TMJ clicking (continuing for more than two years)

Subjects	1988	1989	1990	1991	1992
No. 12 & 18	29.5±2.1	39.5±2.1	39.5±12.0	72.0±19.8	50.5±12.0
Other subjects	30.4±12.5	36.8±17.7	47.1±20.6	46.6±20.0	50.7±27.1
No. 31 & 46	17.0±18.4 †	27.0±21.2	25.5±26.2	17.0±14.1	38.0±31.1
Other subjects	31.5±17.0	40.0±23.2	50.0±27.1	44.0±22.5	52.8±17.1
No. 59 & 60	29.7±10.0	50.7±10.0	46.5±13.4	58.0±0	49.0±11.3
Other subjects	43.8±8.6	52.6±17.7	56.6±22.0	62.8±31.4	75.3±31.3

† $P < 0.005$: significant.

Table 5: Number of filled (T1), decayed (T2) and total number of filled and/or decayed (T1 + T2) teeth of subjects with or without persistent TMJ clicking (continuing for more than two years)

Subjects	T1, T2, T1+ T2	1988	1989	1990	1991	1992
No. 12 & 18	T1	4.0±0	n.r.	3.5±2.1	8.0±1.4	1.0±1.4
	T2	7.5±0.7	n.r.	7.0±2.8	2.5±3.5	1.0±1.4
	T1 + T2	11.5±0.7	n.r.	10.5±4.9	10.5±4.9	2.0±0
Other Subjects	T1	2.5±2.8	n.r.	5.6±3.5	7.3±4.0	3.0±2.1
	T2	3.2±4.1	n.r.	2.6±3.4	1.0±1.0	0.2±0.5
	T1 + T2	5.7±5.2	n.r.	8.5±5.2	8.3±4.5	3.3±1.8
No. 31 & 46	T1	3.0±4.2	n.r.	0	7.5±2.1	1.0±1.4
	T2	7.5±7.8	n.r.	6.0±8.5	3.5±4.9	3.5±4.9
	T1 + T2	10.5±3.5	n.r.	6.0±8.5	11.0±2.8	4.5±3.5
Other Subjects	T1	3.6±2.9	n.r.	5.5±3.0	6.6±3.5	2.6±2.1
	T2	3.6±3.4	n.r.	1.7±2.3	1.0±1.2	1.2±1.9
	T1 + T2	7.4±3.9	n.r.	7.2±3.6	7.7±3.6	3.8±2.7
No. 59 & 60	T1	2.0±0	n.r.	2.5±2.1	3.0±1.4	5.5±0.7
	T2	2.0±0	n.r.	1.5±2.1	2.5±2.1	0.5±0.7
	T1+ T2	4.0±0	n.r.	4.0±0	5.5±0.7	6.0±0
Other Subjects	T1	2.2±1.8	n.r.	3.4±1.9	3.4±1.1	3.8±1.6
	T2	2.7±2.8	n.r.	1.1±1.6	1.1±1.4	0.7±0.8
	T1+ T2	5.0±2.9	n.r.	4.5±2.0	5.5±0.7	4.6±1.9

n.r.= not registered.

In subjects less than 10 years of age, the dentition is generally a mixture of deciduous and permanent teeth. During the mixed dentition stage, numerous occlusal interferences are present and the muscles must repeatedly learn new patterns of mandibular closure to avoid interfering or decayed teeth. The pathway of centric relation (muscular centric position), having only been established in the central nervous system for a short time, is not as entrenched as it is in adults. No repeatedly used position of occlusal contact that does not coincide with the centric relation is ever acquired by chance. Consequently, a discrepancy between the habitual occlusal position and the muscular centric position (bite plate-induced occlusal position) emerges, resulting in temporary clicking. Torii and Chiwata reported a significant relationship between the occlusal discrepancy and TMJ sounds (Torii K & Chiwata I, 2005). In Torii's longitudinal study, as no relationships were observed between persistent clicking and the number of decayed, filled or totaly decayed and filled teeth, the avoidance of decayed or filled teeth was not thought to be a cause of the occlusal discrepancy. These results suggest that persistent clicking was not caused by iatrogenic factors. Generally, teeth that erupt in a malposition that does not coincide with the centric relation may have been repositioned into the correct position coinciding with the centric relation by muscular force; that is the bite force. Under conditions in which an occlusal discrepancy exists until the tooth is repositioned into the correct position, temporary clicking may be produced. However, if the bite force is small before the completion of the permanent dentition, the malposition of occlusion will be maintained. Once the permanent dentition stage has been reached, usually at an age of 10-12 years, the muscles frequently adopt an occlusal position that does not coincide with the muscular centric relation. This new position of occlusal contact usually begins as an expedient process to avoid interferences, providing better function than the centric relation provides at that moment. The continued presence of the occlusal discrepancy causes the new reflex pattern of the pathway to be used so repeatedly that the new position of the mandible may resemble the centric relation (Moyers RE, 1956). In Torii's study, subjects No. 31 and 46 had a significantly smaller bite force at the ages 8 and 9 years, respectively (mixed dentition); thus, occlusal discrepancy may have appeared as a result of the small bite force and this discrepancy may have been maintained once the permanent dentition was achieved, resulting in the persistent clicking. Although no data on the occlusal force at the ages of 8 and 9 years were available for subjects No. 59 and 60, the bite force of these subjects was tend to be smaller than those of the other subjects at later stage (difference not significant; see Table **4**). Therefore, persistent clicking in these subjects was thought to have been caused by an occlusal discrepancy that emerged as a result of small bite force during mixed-dentition stage. For individuals with persistent clicking, examiner in charge of routine dental and oral health examination should tell the subject to visit a dental clinic if TMJ locking or other TMD symptoms appear. If left untreated, these symptoms of TMD may result in irreversible pathologic conditions as will be explained in Chapters 7 and 8. Temporary clicking in Torii's study means that the occlusal discrepancy temporally existed at the eruption of the permanent tooth, but it disappeared with repositioning of the tooth by muscular forces.

4. PREVALENCE IN JAPANESE CHILDREN AND ADOLESCENTS

The prevalence of symptoms and signs of TMDs has been reported in Table **3** from Japan School Dentist Association in 2010. Although the relationship between malocclusion and TMJ dysfunction has not been cleared, morphological malocclusion and TMJ clicking or deviating opening path were recorded.

Table 6: Results of routine dental examination in Japanese kindergarten, elementary school, junior high school and high school in 2010

Boys			**Girls**	**(%)**
	Malocclusion	**TMJ Dysfunction**	**Malocclusion**	**TMJ Dysfunction**
Kindergarten	2.82	0.06	3.57	0.06
Elementary School	4.49	0.16	4.90	0.20
Junior High School	5.37	0.46	5.62	0.57
High School	3.81	0.52	4.44	0.68

The number of school children and adolescents in 2005 included 1,827,534 boys and 1,777,708 girls. The percentages of TMJ dysfunction increased with age in both boys and girls. These data are consistent with the data of the studies in Scandinavian countries. On the other hand, the number of TMD patients in Japan was reported from the Ministry of Health, Labor and Welfare; in June, 2010, the number of newly visited patients was 34,307; patients receiving continued treatment were 49,849. The main treatment modality was appliance therapy. The joint-related TMD (arthrogenous) is thought to need an early treatment to avoid irreversible pathologic change that may occur if it is left untreated. The cases that needed an early treatment are described in the following paragraphs.

Case 1:

This patient was 17 years old, high school student. She visited us with chief complaint of the right TMJ pain and clicking sound in opening mouth and had been aware of TMJ clicking since 12 years of age. The patient's previous medical/dental history was unremarkable. She had been diagnosed as having bilateral disc displacement with reduction of arthralgia.

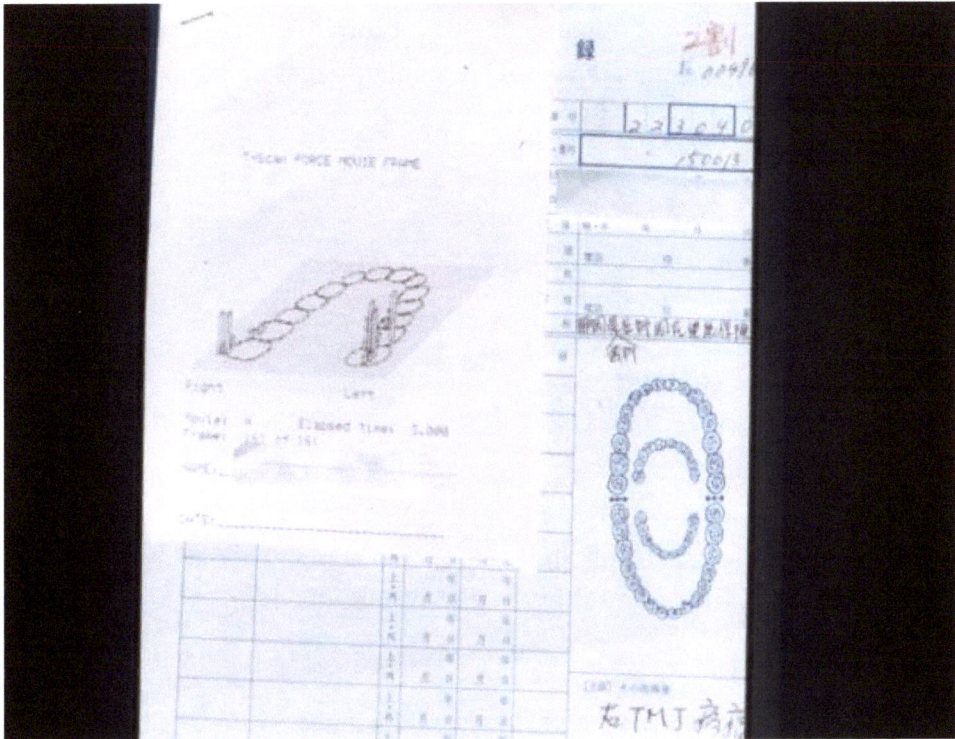

Figure 1: Premature contacts on both second molars.

The treatment procedure is given as follows:

1. First examination was done on March 23, 1993. Impressions were taken for fabricating a full coverage type occlusal splint.

2. On 30th March, the patient wore the splint.

3. On 1st April, her pain relieved and the BPOP (bite plate-induced occlusal position) wax records were taken and the dental casts were then mounted on an articulator. An occlusal analysis was performed and indicated premature occlusal contacts on both second molars (Fig. **1**).

4. Four times of occlusal adjustments in the BPOP were performed. The clicking and pain of the TMJ disappeared in total five weeks of

treatment period. No recurrence has occurred till now. The causal mechanism of this patient's TMD is similar to that in Fig. **2**.

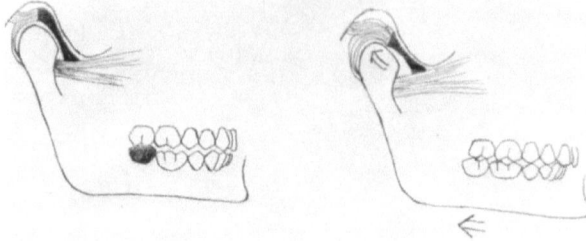

Figure 2: Mechanism of TMJ disc displacement.

Premature occlusal contacts on the second molars make the mandible move posteriorly to meet the teeth, resulting in disc displacement of TMJ.

Case 2:

This patient was 15 years old, junior high school student. He visited us with chief complaints of difficulty of opening mouth and pain in the right TMJ together with other symptoms of fullness of right ear, headache and stiffness of his shoulder. Similar to case 1, an occlusal splint was fabricated and the splint was worn, and then an occlusal analysis was performed. The analysis indicated premature contacts on both molars. Occlusal adjustments were performed in the muscular contact position (BPOP) four times on both the second, the first molars, and on the first and second premolars during two months. His symptoms completely disappeared and did not recur (see Chapter 7).

From these cases, it can be concluded that arthrogenous TMD should be treated early in adolescents.

SUMMARY

Severe symptoms of TMDs in adolescents were rare in previous epidemiological and longitudinal studies. At present, it is unclear whether other moderate TMD symptoms should be left untreated or not.

REFERENCES

Agerberg G & Carlsson GE (1972). Functional disorders of the masticatory system. I. Distribution of symptoms according to age and sex as judged from investigation by questionnaire. *Acta Odontol Scand* 1972;30:597-613.

Ahlberg J, Savolainen A, Rantala M Lindholm H, Könnönen M (2004). Reported bruxism and biopsychosocial symptoms: a longitudinal study. *Community Dent Oral Epidemiol* 2004;32307-311.

De Boever JA, Van den Berghe L (1987). Longitudinal study of functional condition in the masticatory system in Flemish children. *Community Dent Oral Epidemiol* 1987;15:100-103.

De Kanter RJAM, Käyser AF, Battistuzzi PGFCM, Truin GJ, Van'T Hof MA (1992). Demand and need for treatment of craniomandibular dysfunction in Dutch adult population. *J Dent Res* 1992;71:1607-1612

Egermark-Eriksson I, Carlsson GE, Ingervall B (1981). Prevalence of mandibular dysfunction and orofacial parafunction in 7-, 11- and 15-year-old Swedish children. *Eur J Orthod* 1981;3:163-172.

Egermark-Eriksson I (1982). Mandibular dysfunction in children and individuals with dual bite. *Swed Dent J* 1982;Suppl 10:1-45.

Egermark I, Carlsson GE, Magnusson T (2001). A 20-year longitudinal study of subjective symptoms of temporomandibular disorders from children to adulthood. *Acta Odontol Scand* 2001;59:40-48.

Hansson T & Nilner M (1975). A study of the occurrence of symptoms of diseases of the temporomandibular joint masticatory musculature and related structures. *J Oral Rehabil* 1975;2:313324.

Heikinheimo K, Salmi K, Myllärniemi S, Kirveskari P (1989). Symptoms of craniomandibular disorder in a sample of Finnish adolescents at the ages of 12 and 15 years. *Eur J Orthod* 1989;11:325-331.

Helkimo M (1974). Studies on function and dysfunction of masticatory system. I. An epidemiological investigation of symptoms of dysfunction in Lapps in the North Finland. *Proc Finn Dent Soc* 1974;70:37-49.

Helkimo M (1974). Studies on function and dysfunction of the masticatory system. II. Index for anamnestic and clinical dysfunction and occlusal state. *Swed Dent J* 1974;67:101-121.

Helkimo M (1974). Studies on function and dysfunction of the masticatory system. III. Analyses of anamnestic and clinical recordings of dysfunction with the aid of indices. *Swed Dent J* 1974;67:165-182.

Helkimo M (1974). Studies on function and dysfunction of the masticatory system. IV. Age and sex distribution of symptoms of dysfunction of the masticatory system in Lapps in the north of Finland. *Acta Odontol Scand* 1974;32:255-267.

Heft MW (1984). Prevalence of TMJ signs and symptoms in the elderly. *Gerodontology* 1984;3:125-130.

Könönen M, Nyström M, Kleemola-Kujala E, Kataja M, Evälahti M, Laine P, Peck L (1987). Signs nd symptoms of craniomandibular disorders in a series of Finnish children. *Acta Odontol Scand* 1987;45:109-114.

Könönen M & Nyström M (1993). A longitudinal study of craniomandibular disorders in Finnish adolescents. *J Orofac Pain* 1993;7:329-336.

Köhler AA, Helkimo AN, Magnusson T, Hugoson A (2009). Prevalence of symptoms and signs indicative of temporomandibular disorders in children and adolescents. A cross-sectional epidemiological investigation covering two decades. *Eur Arch Paediatr Dent* 2009;10 (Suppl. 1):16-25.

Lipton JA, Ship JA, Larach-Robinson D (1993). Estimated prevalence and distribution of reported orofacial pain in the United States. *J Am Dent Assoc* 1993:115-121.

Macfarlane TV, Blinkhorn AS, Davies RM, Kincey J, Worthington HV (2004). Predictors of outcome for orofacial pain in the general population: a four-year follow-up study. *J Dent Res* 2004;83:712-717.

Magnusson T, Egermark-Eriksson I, Carlsson GE (1985). Four-year longitudinal study of mandibular dysfunction in children. *Community Dent Oral Epidemiol* 1985;13:117-120.

Magnusson T, Egermark-Eriksson I, Carlsson GE (1986). Five-year longitudinal study of signs and symptoms of mandibular dysfunction in adolescents. *J Craniomandib Pract* 1986;4:339-343.

Magnusson T, Egermark I, Carlsson GE (2000). A longitudinal epidemiologic study of signs and symptoms of temporomandibular disorders from 15 to 35 years of age. *J Orofac Pain* 2000;14:310-319.

Marklund S & Wänman A (2008). Incidence and prevalence of myofascial pain in the jaw-face region. A one-year prospective study on dental students. *Acta Odonotol Scand* 2008;66:113-121.

Moyers RE (1956). Some physiologic considerations of centric and other jaw relations. *J Prosthet Dent* 1956;6:183-194.

Nilner M & Lassing S (1981). Prevalence of functional disturbances and disease of the stomatognathic system in 7-14 year olds. *Swed Dent J* 1981;5:173-187.

Nilner M (1981). Prevalence of functional disturbances and disease of the stomatognathic system in 15-18 year olds. *Swed Dent J* 1981;5:189-197.

Nilsson I (2007). Reliability, validity, incidence and impact of temporomandibular pain and disorders in adolescents [Thesis]. *Swed Dent J* 2007; Suppl. 183:1-85.

Rammelsberg P, LeResche L, Dworkin S, Mancl L (2003). Longitudinal outcome of temporomandibular disorders: a 5-year epidemiological study of muscle disorders defined by research diagnostic criteria for temporomandibular disorders. *J Orofac Pain* 2003;17:9-20.

Rugh JD & Solberg WK (1985). Oral health in the United States: Temporomandibular disorders. *J Dent Educ* 1985;49:398-404.

Thilander B, Rubio G, Pena L, Mayorga C (2002). Prevalence of temporomandibular dysfunction and its association with malocclusion in children and adolescents: An epidemiologic study related to specified stage of dental development. *Angl Orthod* 2002;72:146-154.

Torii K & Chiwata I (2005). Relationship between habitual occlusal position and flat bite plane-induced occlusal position in volunteers with and without temporomandibular joint sounds. *Cranio* 2005;23:16-21.

Torii K (2011). Longitudinal course of temporomandibular joint sounds in Japanese children and adolescents. *Head & Face Medicine* 2011, 7:17, Available from http://www.head-face-med.com/content/7/1/17

Wahlund K (2003). Temporomandibular disorders in adolescents. Epidemiological and methodological studies and a randomized controlled trial [thesis]. *Swed Dent J* 2003; Supp. 164:1-64.

Wänman A (1987). Craniomandibular disorders in adolescents. A longitudinal study in an urban Swedish population [thesis]. *Swed Dent J* 1987; Suppl. 44:1-61.

Wänman A & Agerberg G (1991). Etiology of craniomandibular disorders: evaluation of some occlusal and psychosocial factors in 19-year-olds. *J Craniomandib Disord* 1991;5:35-44.

Wänman A (1996). Longitudinal course of symptoms of craniomandibular disorders in men and women. A 10-year follow-up study of an epidemiologic sample. *Acta Odontol Scand* 1996;54:337-342.

Widmalm SE, Christiansen RL, Gunn SM, Haley LM (1995). Prevalence of signs and symptoms of craniomandibular disorders and orofacial parafunction in 4-6-year-old African-American and Caucasian children. *J Oral Rehabil* 1995;22:87-93.

CHAPTER 2

Causes and Contributing Factors of Temporomandibular Disorders

Abstract: Various contributing factors for temporomandibular disorders have been enumerated; occlusal factors, trauma, habits (bruxism, lip-, tongue-, and nail-biting) and psychological factors. However, prominent factors have not been found.

Keywords: Occlusion, habits, trauma, contributing factors, grinding, clenching, myofascial pain, muscle tenderness, headache, occlusal interferences, osteoarthrosis, clicking, crepitation, malocclusion, psychological factor.

1. INTRODUCTION

It is clear that TMDs have been originally thought to be caused by occlusal interferences, because initial studies of TMDs were especially carried out in Europe, and performed to relate occlusal factors and TMDs. However, since the occlusal factors had not been related to TMDs, other contributing factors have been sought. Initially, parafunctions, such as grinding and clenching of the teeth, biting of the cheek, lip and tongue, and nail biting were suspected as aggravating factors. In addition, traumatic factors have been included in contributing factors of TMDs. However, the causes of TMDs have essentially been thought to be in structural variables of human except trauma, therefore, many epidemiological studies have been performed in children and adolescents.

2. OCCLUSAL FACTORS

Butler *et al.* surveyed patients with myofascial pain syndrome and asymptomatic patients and reported that analysis of static and functional relationship did not reveal a significant difference between patients with jaw dysfunction and asymptomatic patients, and they summarized that signs and symptoms associated with the myofascial pain-dysfunction syndrome (MPD) were observed and tabulated in 56 patients ranging from 16 to 73 years of age. Many patients were aware of bruxism habits, and a history of gastrointestinal tract disturbances was common. Eighty-four percent of the patients were women which suggested that myofascial pain to be linked with sex. The patients with MPD commonly complained of muscle tenderness to palpation particularly associated with masseter, temporal, lateral and medial pterygoid muscles. Headache was associated with muscle symptoms, especially tenderness of the anterior temporal muscle (Butler JH *et al.*, 1975). Kopp compared 20 patients with TMJ-crepitation (E_1-group) and 19 patients with TMJ palpatory tenderness (E_2-group) with 29 other patients with mandibular dysfunction (R-group), and reported that no statistically significant differences could be found between groups with respect to clinical signs, occlusal interferences or dental attrition. Loss of molar support was found to be significantly more frequent in the E_1-group than in the R-group. And Kopp described that molar loss played a role in the etiology of TMJ osteoarthrosis (Kopp S, 1977). Helöe and Helöe investigated the occurrence of TMJ-disorders in an elderly population (241 persons aged 65-79) and reported that eight per cent of the group had had TMJ pain recently, and fourteen per cent reported to have said had clicking or crepitation. These symptoms were twice as commonly reported by women as men and they were also most frequent among people complaining of rheumatism or general joint pain. By clinical examination, clicking and/or crepitation was found in 27% of the individuals. They described that dental/prosthetic status had seemingly no distinct influence on the symptoms since 92% of the participants wore dentures (Helöe B & Helöe LA, 1977). Mohlin *et al.* studied the relation between malocclusion, symptoms of mandibular dysfunction and cuspal interferences in 389 men aged 21-54 years and reported that crossbite was found to be related to mandibular dysfunction only when general factors were kept constant and described that the results of their study also suggest a multifactorial aetiology of madibular pain and dysfunction (Mohlin B *et al.*, 1980). De Boever and Adriaens investigated a group of 135 patients (thirty-three males and 102 females) seeking treatment for pain dysfunction of the TMJ and reported that no real pattern in the occurrence of the type of prematurity relative to the severity of the dysfunction could be observed and no correlation could be found between the severity of the symptoms and the number of occluding pairs of premolars and molars: $r=-0.03$. However, after the treatments (reassurance, occlusal splint, muscle exercise and occlusal adjustment), the correlation coefficient between the treatment results (expressed as the decrease in dysfunction points) and the number of occluding molars and premolars was

r=0.47 after 6 months and r=0.51 after 12 months (De Boever JA & Adriaens PA, 1983). Roberts *et al.* examined 205 patients with TMJ symptoms (222 joints, 188 unilateral and 17 bilateral) clinically and arthrographicall for TMJ internal derangements and divided them into three arthrographic groups as "normal", showing "meniscus displacement with reduction", or showing "meniscus displacement without reduction". They reported that no significant differences were found between arthrographic groups with respect to Angle classification, horizontal and vertical overlap, posterior tooth wear, missing posterior teeth, cuspid-protected occlusion, balancing-side contacts, deflective occlusion and clenching of the teeth, and tilted teeth on the contralateral side were more common in case of reducing meniscal dislocation than in case of normal meniscus position or of nonreducing meniscus dislocation (Roberts CA *et al.*, 1987). Gunn *et al.* examined 151 migrant children, aged 6 to 18 years and reported that malocclusion parameter exhibited by the largest number of subjects was excessive overbite (45.7%), and the most frequently found clinical symptoms were muscle pain on chewing (22.5%) and noises near ears (20.0%). Clinical and reported signs and symptoms did not, in this population, appear to be related to malocclusion (Gunn SM *et al.*, 1988). On the other hand, since Krogh-Poulsen and Olsson described "that the retruded contact position (RCP) is the most cranial position of the mandible after it has performed a terminal hinge closure. A short, straightforward slide from the RCP into the intercuspal position (ICP) seems to be a harmonious pattern in most human dentitions, both in adults and children. However, interferences which cause the mandible to slide from the RCP into the ICP through an oblique course from symmetrical movement are commonly considered a cause of functional disturbances of the stomatognathic system". Many researchers have investigated the relationship between these interferences in the RCP, or slide from the RCP into the ICP and TMDs (Krogh-Poulsen WG & Olsson A, 1966). Geering reported that a slide in combination with balancing interference was found almost twice as frequently in patients with pain and/or symptoms compared to patients with no symptoms. Neither the amount nor the direction of the slide was correlated with the pain and/or symptoms. It was also reported that the balancing interferences tend to be located on the pain and/or symptom side (Geering AH 1974). Ingervall *et al.* investigated 389 Swedish men (median age 32 years) and reported that impaired chewing function was noted in about 10%, different types of parafunction in 26%, frequent headaches in 5%, TMJ or muscle pain in 3% and difficulties in mouth opening in 10% of the men, and locking or luxation of the mandible was the most prevalent clinical symptom (24%), followed by reduced movement capacity and deviation on opening of the mandible, TMJ-sounds and muscle tenderness. Sixty per cent of the men had one or more clinical symptoms of dysfunction. In addition, they reported that positive correlations were found between subjective symptoms of dysfunction and non-working side interference as well as single tooth contact on the working side, and muscle tenderness was positively correlated with interferences in the retruded position of the mandible (Ingervall B *et al.*, 1980). Nilner and Lassing performed an epidemiological investigation in 440 Swedish children (7-14 year olds) and reported that the interview revealed 36% with symptoms, 15% with recurrent headaches and 13% reported clicking sounds from TMJ; 77% of the children reported at least one of the following oral parafunctions: grinding, clenching, lip- and cheek-biting or thumb-sucking. They also described that occlusal interferences in retruded position (RP) were found in 79 % and mediotrusion interferences (balancing contacts) in 78 %, and more than half of the children approx. 64%, claimed pain on palpation of the temporomandibular joint muscles and more than one third (39%) claimed pain on palpation of the TMJ. However, they did not relate these interferences to TMD symptoms (Nilner M & Lassing S, 1981). Egermark-Eriksson reported that 60 % of 402 Swedish school children (7-, 11, and 15 years) had some form of occlusal anomaly and most of the children (60%) had an RP-IP (retruded contact position-intercuspal position) displacement of 0.5-1.0 mm antero-posteriorly while 1% had dual bite (Egermark-Eriksson, 1982). Nilner interviewed 749 children and adolescents and examined their occlusion and reported that correlations were found in the older age group (age range 15 to 18 years) between interferences in RP (retruded position) and deviation at maximal mouth opening ($p<0.01$), tenderness to palpation of the TMJ laterally ($p<0.05$) and between unilateral interferences in RP and irregular movements and deviations at maximal opening ($p<0.01$). The masseter muscle and the attachment of the temporal muscle were tender on palpation more often in adolescents with mediotrusion interferences (balancing side contacts) than in young people without mediotrusion interferences ($p<0.05$) (Nilner M, 1986). Helkimo investigated Lapps in the North of Finland on function and dysfunction of the masticatory system. He described that no attempts were made to compare the anamnestic and clinical dysfunction index, because none of the individuals filled the requirements of index value zero, and he said the index for occlusal state which was designed in accordance with well established principles for "ideal occlusion" is apparently unrealistic, at any rate for this population (Helkimo M, 1974). Könönen *et al.* investigated the prevalences of subjective symptoms and clinical signs of craniomandibular disorders (CMD) in a series of Finnish children (n=166) and reported that 52 % of the children reported at least one subjective symptom, and 75% at least one parafunctional habit, and clinical signs were common but rarely severe in accordance with Helkimo's clinical dysfunction index, and both the number of subjective symptoms (p<0.001) and the number of orofacial parafunctions (p<0.05) correlated with the clinical dysfunction index. They also reported that 42 % of the children had at least one of the interferences (unilarteral contact in RP (retruded position) and other interferences in mediotrusion, laterotrusion, or protrusion) (Könönen M *et al.*, 1987). Egermark-Eriksson concluded from the dual bite study that (1) the clinically measured antero-posterior distance between RP and IP (intercuspal position) varied between 2.5 and 5.0 mm, with a mean of 3.9, and in some individuals, occlusal wear was excessive. Four subjects reported subjective symptoms and the clinical signs of dysfunction according to Helkimo were judged to be absent or mild in 7 subjects, moderate in 4 and severe in 1 subject; (2) in the electromyographic study, it was found that neither of the two mandibular positions (IP and RP or close to RP) gave a balanced activity in the anterior and posterior temporal muscles or in the masseter muscles during maximal bite. The duration of the muscle activity in the individual chewing cycles was longer in the subjects with dual bite than in the controls (the antero-posterior distance between RP and IP was 0-1 mm); (3) the pattern of muscle activity during chewing indicated that the retruded mandibular position was also used during chewing. It therefore seems logical to create a stable occlusion in or close to RP in patients with dual bite (Egermark-Erikson I, 1982, b). In addition, it was concluded from the epidemiological study that (1) Nocturnal tooth grinding was reported by 20% of 7-year-olds and 10 % of 11- and 15-year-olds. Twenty per cent of the youngest children and 3 % of 11-year-olds reported finger-sucking. Children with prolonged sucking habit more often had frontal open bite and crossbite than children without this habit; (2) One or more of the symptoms of mandibular dysfunction (TMJ sounds, tiredness in the jaws and face and difficulties in mouth opening) were reported by 16-25 % of the children. The symptoms were mostly occasional and only three children had frequent symptoms. Twenty-three per cent of the children reported recurrent headache, *i.e.* headache once a month or more often; (3) Muscle tenderness on palpation (33%) and TMJ sounds (18%) were the most common clinical signs of mandibular dysfunction, increasing with age. Mild dysfunction was very common, while moderate or severe dysfunction was found in 4, 8 and 14 % of 7-, 11- and 15-year-old children, respectively; (4) Sixty per cent of the children had morphological malocclusion, 73 % had functional malocclusion and 1 % dual bite; (5) Children who reported subjective symptoms of dysfunction and recurrent headache more often had clinical signs of mandibular dysfunction than children without these symptoms. In addition, those children who had mandibular dysfunction also had more worn teeth than other children; (6) Functional malocclusion or occlusal interference seems to be more important than morphological malocclusion in explaining the existence of mandibular dysfunction. However, morphological malocclusion such as postnormal occlusion, prenormal occlusion, frontal open bite and crossbite may predispose to functional malocclusion and thus secondarily to mandibular dysfunction; and (7) In the stepwise multiple regression analysis, the correlations found were numerically weak. Four of the examined variables (two different types of occlusal interferences, age and psychological qualities) were more important other variables in explaining the variance of the clinical dysfunction index. The etiology of mandibular dysfunction in children seems to be multifactorial (Egermark-Eriksson I, 1982, a). Wänman performed a longitudinal study on 17-year-old adolescents during three years and concluded that (1) Signs and symptoms of mandibular dysfunction were commonly reported and mostly mild; (2) Girls reported symptoms more often than boys at the age of 18 and 19; (3) Muscle tenderness on palpation and TMJ sounds were the most common signs. Girls had signs of mandibular dysfunction more often than boys; (4) Signs and symptoms of mandibular dysfunction fluctuated longitudinally; (5) There was a positive relationship between signs and symptoms of mandibular dysfunction; (6) Oral parafunction was commonly reported. Reports of occlusal ones such as clenching and grinding of teeth increased during the study period, while reports of orofacial parafunctions such as nail-, lip, cheek-, and tongue-biting decreased; (7) About one third of the adolescents had morphological malocclusion. Of the functional malocclusion recorded, unilateral contact in RP varied most between the recordings. About one fifth had a lateral slide between RP and IP and about 30% had mediotrusion interferences; (8) The occurrence of mediotrusive interferences was the only occlusal variable that was partly related to some signs of mandibular dysfunction. Those weak correlations and the fluctuating symptoms support the view of a multifactorial etiology; (9) Recurrent headaches were reported three times more often by girls than boys. Girls also reported more intense headache than boys; (10) A positive relationship was found between recurrent headaches and signs and symptoms of mandibular dysfunction; (11) A smaller group had signs and symptoms of mandibular dysfunction during the whole studied period. Since these may be at a greater risk in the development of signs and symptoms of mandibular dysfunction, additional longitudinal studies are needed; and (12) The results in the present study indicate that a stomatognathic examination should be included in the routine dental check-ups to evaluate the frequency, intensity and duration of craniomandibular disorders, even though the need and demand for treatment may be small in adolescents (Wänman A, 1987). Conti *et al.* performed a cross-sectional study on students in high school and university and reported that a total of 0.65% of the subjects had severe TMD symptoms, 5.81% had moderate symptoms and 34.84% had mild symptoms. Those with severe and moderate symptom levels were interpreted to be in need of treatment. Symptoms were found significantly more frequently in females than in males. Self-reported emotional tension and parafunctional habits demonstrated strong associations with TMD ($p<0.01$). Occlusion did not seem to influence the presence or severity of TMD. Based on these results, the efficacy of some traditional TMD treatments should be reconsidered, and reversible and conservative procedures should be the first choice for managing TMD patients (Conti PCR *et al.*, 1996). From the studies regarding RCP analysis, the relationship between occlusal factors and TMDs remains unclear. Therefore, the studies on occlusal adjustments in RCP have been performed where will be described in Chapter 3. On the other hand, Marklund and Wänman investigated dental students during 1-year period and reported that the 1-year period prevalence of frequent myofascial symptoms was 19%. The incidence of myofascial pain was 4%. Female students presented an almost 4-fold incidence rate of myofascial symptoms compared to the male students. They measured mandibular stability in the ICP if the molar teeth could keep a firm grip on a foil during moderate clenching and concluded that both self-reported bruxism and registered mandibular instability in ICP showed association with 1-year period prevalence of myofascial signs and symptoms in the jaw-face region (Marklund S & Wänman A, 2008).

Türp *et al.* described that one important outcome of the modern understanding of occlusion should be avoidance of occlusion-changing procedures in healthy functioning patients, while another should be the recognition that irreversible treatments are rarely required in the treatment of orofacial pain patients. (Türp JC *et al.*, 2008). On the other hand, Slavicek described that the functions of the masticatory organ are entirely different and closely networked with somatic and psychic functions of the brain (Slavicek R, 2011). Regarding the relation of occlusion with TMDs, Manfredini *et al.* described as follows: There is no evidence for the existence of a predictable relationship between occlusal and postural features and it is clear that the presence of TMD pain is not related to the existence of measurable occluso-postural abnormalities. Therefore, the use instruments and techniques aiming to measure purported occlusal, electromyographic, kinesiographic or posturographic abnormalities cannot be justified in the evidence-based TMD practice (Manfredini D *et al.*, 2012).

3. PARAFUNCTIONS

Agerberg and Carlsson investigated 1106 persons (15-74 year old) regarding TMDs and reported that orofacial parafunction (the habit of grinding teeth, pressing teeth together, biting tongue or cheek or lips or nails, or anything else) and TMJ sounds were most closely correlated with functional pain (Agerberg G & Carlsson GE, 1973). Zarb and Thompson examined 194 patients with TMJ pain dysfunction syndrome and reported that 47 patients had bruxism (Zarb GA & Thompson GW, 1975). Moss *et al.* reported that nocturnal bruxism was found to be self-reported at a significantly higher frequency in combination with TMJ and jaw muscle pain group compared to the No facial pain and TMJ pain group (Moss RA *et al.*, 1984). Wänman reported that habits of oral parafunction such as grinding and clenching were related to the frequency of headache (p<0.001) but not the intensity (Wänman A, 1987). Magnusson *et al.* performed a longitudinal study of signs and symptoms of TMDs on 15-year-old subjects (135) at intervals of 5, 10, and 20 years and reported that there was a substantial fluctuation of both reported symptoms and clinically recorded signs over the 20-year period, but progression to severe pain and dysfunction of the masticatory system was rare in both the 15-year-old and 35-year-old subjects and 13% reported 1 or more frequent TMD symptoms. At age 35, only 3 subjects (3%) were classified as having severe or moderate clinical signs of dysfunction according to the Helkimo Index. Women reported TMD symptoms and headache and had muscle tenderness and joint sounds more often than men. Correlation between the studied variables was mainly weak. The highest correlation ($r_s = 0.4$) was between reported clenching and bruxing habits and TMJ sounds and jaw fatigue (Magnusson T *et al.* 2000). Manfredini *et al.* performed a cross-sectional study on the prevalence of bruxism in subjects with and without TMDs and reported that a significant association between bruxism and TMDs emerged ($p<0.05$). The highest prevalence of bruxism was found in patients with the following diagnoses: combined myofascial pain and disk displacement (87.5%); combined myofascial pain, disk displacement and other joint conditions (73.3%); and myofascial pain (68.9%). They described from the results of their study that bruxism has stronger relationship with muscle disorders than with disk displacement and joint pathologies, and such relationship seems to be independent of the presence of other RDC/TMD diagnosis along with myofascial pain (Manfredini D *et al.*, 2003). Dao *et al.* compared pain and quality of life in bruxers (19 nocturnal bruxers) and patients with myofascial pain (61 patients with no evidence of bruxism) and reported that pain was more intense in those bruxers who reported pain than among the myofascial pain patients, even though pain was not the chief complaint of bruxers. Both conditions reduced the patient's quality of life, although pain patients (either bruxism or myofascial pain) appeared to be much more affected than bruxers who were pain-free. They described that the fact that pain from bruxism was worst in the morning suggests that it is possibly a form of post exercise muscle soreness, and that myofascial pain, which was worst late in the day, is likely to have a different etiology (Dao TTT *et al.*, 1994). On the other hand, Pergamalian *et al.* investigated the association between wear facets, bruxism and severity of facial pain in patients with TMDs and reported that tooth wear was modestly correlated with age, but bruxism was not associated with the amount of wear and bruxism activity was not correlated with muscle pain on palpation and inversely associated with TMJ pain on palpation (Pergamalian A *et al*., 2003). Although many studies regarding the relationship between parafunction and TMD have been published, the conclusion has still not been drawn (Pullinger AG & Seligman DA, 1993; Manfredini D *et al*., 2003; Hirsh C *et al*., 2004; Schierz O *et al*., 2007; Nagamatsu-Sakaguchi C *et al*., 2008; Fernandes G *et al*., 2013).

4. TRAUMA

Zarb and Thompson reported patients having history of trauma (trauma related to dental or medical procedures: 5 patients; trauma from biting into hard foods, excessive yawning, blows or whiplash: 6 patients) (Zarb GA & Thompson GW., 1975). Pullinger and Seligman investigated the association of trauma history with TMDs among six diagnostic subgroups of 230 patients (DD: disk displacement with reduction; DD: disk displacement without reduction; OA: osteoarthrosis with prior derangement history; OA: primary OA; myalgia; subluxation only) and reported that except for subluxation (29%), trauma history typified TMD patient groups 1 to 5 (63%, 79%, 44%, 53%, 54%) (p<0.001) compared to 13% and 18% of asymptomatic and symptomatic control subjects, and 11% of general dental patients. The high prevalence of trauma in the myalgia-only group complicates the concept of myofascial pain-dysfunction syndrome as solely a stress or centrally mediated disorder. DD without reduction (43%) and with reduction (38%) had the highest prevalence of motor vehicle accident trauma, myalgia and OA groups had prevalence while less subluxation-only cases had none. On the other hand, patients with DD without reduction were also the only group to report multiple trauma (29%), suggesting that although specific traumatic events may seem to precipitate clinical symptoms, they may not always have initiated the problem. Trauma may be both an important cumulative and precipitating event in TMDs (Pullinger AG & Seligman DA, 1991). Steed and Wexler compared presenting symptoms and treatment outcomes in patients suffering from TMD as a result of traumatic *versus* nontraumatic etiology. They described that for traumatic group, the reported length of the TMD problem was of shorter duration when compared to the nontraumatic patient group. Trauma patients reported significantly higher percentages of improvement in palpation pain and perceived malocclusion. No significant differences were found for pain report, joint dysfunction, stress, and TMD symptomatology, as measured by the TMJ Scale's Global domain. They concluded that trauma patients manifest different outcomes from nontrauma patients only in pain, perceived malocclusion and non-TM factors. Improvement in percentages does not differ significantly for overall symptoms, pain report, joint dysfunction or limited mandibular range of motion. These results suggest that part of the disagreement can be traced to inconsistent and unvalidated outcome measures, together with small sample sizes and widely varying treatment modalities. Data from the large multi-site study examined here suggest that trauma patients present with significantly higher levels of some TMD symptoms (no differences were found for joint dysfunction). However, treatment outcomes were unrelated to trauma/untrauma status. This suggests that more sophisticated and validated TMD measurement tools should be used for outcome research by the clinician. Earlier studies which relied upon simple *improved-not improved* determinations, or which relied upon patient behaviors to measure improvement, are clearly inadequate. Additionally, this review tends to support the notion that psychosocial factors in the etiology of TMD may have previously been misinterpreted, and that it is likely, perhaps probable, that physical dysfunction of TMD whether it be traumatically or nontraumatically induced, leads to psychosocial problems, and not the reverse (Steed PA & WexlerGB, 2001). Kasch *et al.* compared 19 acute whiplash patients exposed to a motor vehicle accident involving a rear collision with the control group which consisted of 20 age- and gender-matched ankle-injury patients and concluded that TMD pain after whiplash injury and ankle injury is rare, suggesting that whiplash injury is not a major risk factor in the development of TMD problems (Kasch H *et al.*, 2002). On the other hand, Mikhail and Rosen described that to complete the screening for the etiology of MPD (myofascial-pain dysfunction syndrome), it is essential to eliminate the possibility of medically linked factors, recent major surgical operations, or trauma of the head and neck (such as blow to the jaw or whiplash of the head as could result from automobile accidents or recent airplane trip) which may present signs and symptoms of MPD (Mikhail M & Rosen H, 1980).

5. PSYCHOLOGICAL FACTORS

Rugh described that the experiences of pain and pain behavior are dependent on or modified by host factors including the following: (1) tissue damage, (2) anxiety, (3) depression, (4) perceived control, (5) attention, (6) past history with health care professionals, (7) past experiences with pain, (8) personality characteristics, (9) cultural factors, (10) reinforcement history, and (11) beliefs about pain. In addition, he described that a brief history and oral examinations are insufficient to understand patients with complex oral pain conditions. These patients may be better served by attending to and incorporating the new multidimensional concepts of pain now being employed with other complex pain conditions (Rugh JD, 1987). Gerschman *et al.* compared 130 patients with dental phobias and 368 patients with chronic orofacial pain for psychological and social variables and reported that patients in pain showed a greater burden of psychiatric disorders and were more likely to be older, married, have children, be migrants, be less educated, have poorer jobs and be more financially disadvantaged than phobic patients (Gerschman JA *et al.*, 1987). Kinney *et al.*, interviewed 50 chronic TMD patients with DSM-III(R) (the Diagnostic and Statistical Manual of Mental Disorders III) and reported that 46 % of the chronic TMD patients had current Axis I disorders, excluding somatoform pain disorder. They described that professionals who work with chronic TMD patient may need to be aware of and treat the psychological sequelae of these conditions and refer the patient to a psychological evaluation when warranted (Kinney RK *et al.*, 1992).

Maixner *et al.*, described the method of the OPPERA study (Orofacial Pain Prospective Evaluation and Risk Assessment study) (Maixner W *et al.*, 2011). Fillingim *et al.*, performed an OPPERA case-control study and reported that odds of TMD were associated with higher levels of psychosocial symptoms, affective distress, somatic awareness and pain catastrophizing (Fillingim RB *et al.*, 2011).

SUMMARY

Although occlusal factors in TMDs still remain unclear, the research for occlusal factors should be continued, because many occlusal factors that could be related to the development of TMDs have still not been thoroughly evaluated.

REFERENCES

Agerberg G & Carlsson GE (1973). Functional disorders of the masticatory system. II. Symptoms in relation to impaired mobility of the mandible as judged from investigation by questionnaire. *Acta Odontol Scand* 1973;31:335-347.

Butler JH, Folke LE, Bandt CL (1975). A descriptive survey of signs and symptoms associated with the myofascial pain-dysfunction syndrome. *J Am Dent Assoc* 1975;90:635-639.

Conti PCR, Ferreira PM, Pegoraro LF, Conti JV, Salvador MCG (1996). A cross-sectional study of prevalence and etiology of signs and symptoms of temporomandibular disorders in high school and university students. *J Orofac Pain* 1996;10:254-262.

Dao TTT, Lund JP, Lavigne GJ (1994). Comparison of pain and quality of life in bruxers and patients with myofascial pain of the masticatory muscles. *J Orofac Pain* 1994;8:350-356.

De Boever JA & Adriaens PA (1983). Occlusal relationship in patients with pain-dysfunction symptoms in the temporomandibular joints. *J Oral Rehabil* 1983;10:1-7.

Egermark-Eriksson I (1982, a). Mandibular dysfunction in children and in individuals with dual bite. *Swed Dent J* 1982;Suppl. 10:1-45.

Egermark-Eriksson I (1982, b). Malocclusion and some functional recordings of the masticatory system in Swedish school children. *Swed Dent J* 1982;6:9-20.

Fernandes G, Franco AL, Goncalves DA, Speciali JG, Bigal Me, Camparis CM (2013). Temporomandibualr disorders, sleepb ruxism, and primary headaches are mutually associated. *J Orofac Pain* 2013;27:14-20.

Fillingim RB, Ohrbach R, Greenspan JD, Knott C, Dubner R, Bair E, Baraian C, Slade GD, Maixner W (2011). Potential psychosocial risk factors for chronic TMD: descriptive data and empirically identified domains from the OPPERA case-control study. *J Pain* 2011;12 (11 Suppl):T46-60.

Geering AH (1974). Occlusal interferences and functional disturbances of the masticatory system. *J Clin Periodontol* 1974;1:112-119.

Gerschman JA, Wright JL, Hall WD, Read PC, Burrows GD, Holwill BJ (1987). Comparisons of psychological and social factors in patients with chronic oro-facial pain and dental phobic disorders. *Aust Dent J* 1987;32:331-335.

Gunn SM, Woolfolk MW, Faja BW (1988). Malocclusion and TMJ symptoms in migrant children. *J Craniomandib Disord Facial Oral Pain* 1988;2:196-200.

Helöe B & Helöe LA (1977). The occurrence of TMJ-disorders in an elderly population as evaluated by recording of <<subjective>> and <<objective>> symptoms. *Acta Odontol Scand* 1977;36:3 9.

Helkimo M (1974). Studies on function and dysfunction of the masticatory system. II. Index for anamnestic and clinical dysfunction and occlusal state. *Sven Tandlaek Tidskr* 1974a;67:101-119.

Hirsch C, John MT, Schroeder E, Lobbezoo F, Setz JM, Schaller H (2004). Incisal tooth wear and self-reported TMD pain in children and adolescents. *Int J Prosthodont* 2004;17:205-210.

Ingervall B, Mohlin B, Thilander B (1980). Prevalence of symptoms of functional disturbances of the masticatory system in Swedish men. *J Oral Rehabil* 1980;7:185-197.

Karsch H, Hjorth T, Svensson P, Nyhuus L, Jensen TS (2002). Temporomandibular disorders after whiplash injury: A controlled, prospective study. *J Orofac Pain* 2002;16:118-128.

Kinney RK, Gatchel RJ, Ellis E, Holt C (1992). Major psychological disorders in chronic TMD patients : Implications for successful management. *J Am Dent Assoc* 1992;123:49-54.

Könönen M, Nyström M, Kleemola-Kujala E, Kataja M, Evälahti M, Laine P, Peck L (1987). Signs and symptoms of craniomandibular disorders in a series of Finnish children. *Acta Odontol Scand* 1987;45:109-114.

Kopp S (1977). Clinical findings in temporomandibular joint osteoarthrosis. *Scand J Dent Res* 1977;85:434-443.

Krogh-Poulsen WG & Olsson A (1966). Occlusal disharmonies and dysfunction of the stomatognathic system. *Dent Clin North Am* 1966;Nov. :627-635.

Magnusson T, Egermark I, Carlsson GE (2000). A longitudinal epidemiologic study of signs and symptoms of temporomandibular disorders from, 15 to 35 years of age. *J Orofac Pain* 2000;14:310-319.

Maixner W, Diatchenko L, Dubner R, Fillingim RB, Greenspan JD, Knott C, Ohrbach R, Weir B, Slade G (2011). Orofacial Pain Prospective Evaluation and Risk Assessment Study – The OPPERA study. *J Pain* 2011;12 (11 Suppl):T4-T11.

Manfredini D, Cantini E, Romagnoli M Bosco M (2003). Prevalence of bruxism in patient with different research diagnostic criteria for temporomandibular disorders (RDC/TMD) diagnoses. *J Cranio Mandib Pract* 2003;21:279-285.

Manfredini D, Castroflorio T, Perinetti G, Guarda-Nardini L (2012). Dental occlusion, body posture and temporomandibular disorders: where we are now and where we are heading for. *J Oral Rehabil* 2012;39:463-471.

Marklund S & Wänman A (2008). Incidence and prevalence of myofascial pain in the jaw-face region. A one-year prospective study on dental students. *Acta Odontol Scand 2008;66:113-121.*

Mikhail M & Rosen H (1980). History and etiology of myofascial pain-dysfunction syndrome. *J Prosthet Dent* 1980;44:438-444.

Mohlin B, Ingervall B, Thilander B (1980). Relation between malocclusion and mandibular dysfunction in Swedish men. *Eur J Orthod* 1980;2:229-238.

Moss RA, Ruff MM, Sturgis ET (1984). Oral behavioral patterns in facial pain, headache and non-headache populations. *Behav Res Ther* 1984;22:683-687.

Nagamatsu-Sakaguchi C, Minakuchi H, Clark GT, Kuboki T (2008). Relationship between the frequency of sleep bruxism and the prevalence of signs and symptoms of temporomandibular disorders in an adolescent population. *Int J Prosthodont* 2008;21:292-298.

Nilner M, & Lassing S (1981). Prevalence of functional disturbances and diseases of stomatognathic system in 7-14 year olds. *Swed Dent J* 1981;5:173-187.

Nilner M (1986). Functional disturbances and diseases of the stomatognathic system. A cross-sectional study. *J Pedod* 1986;10:211-238.

Pergamalian A, Rudy TE, Zaki HS, Greco CM (2003). The association between wear facets, bruxism, and severity of facial pain in patients with temporomandibular disorders. *J Prosthet Dent* 2003;90:194-200.

Pullinger AG & Seligman DA (1991). Trauma history in diagnostic groups of temporomandibualr disorders. *Oral Surg Oral Med Oral Pathol* 1991;71:529-534.

Pullinger AG & Seligman DA (1993). The degree to which attrition characterizes differentiated patient groups of temporomandibular disorders. *J Orofac Pain* 1993;7:196-208.

Roberts CA, Tallents RH, Katzberg RW, Sanchez-Woodworth RE, Espeland MA, Hadelman SL (1987). Comparison of internal derangements of the TMJ with occlusal findings. *Oral Surg Oral Med Oral Pathol* 1987;63:645-650.

Rugh JD (1987). Psychological components of Pain. *Dent Clin North Am* 1987;31:579-594.

Schierz O, John MT, Schroeder E, Labbezoo F (2007). Association between anterior tooth wear and temporomandibular disorder pain in a German population. *J Prosthet Dent* 2007;97:305-309.

Slavicek R (2011). Relationship between occlusion and temporomandibular disorders: implication for the gnathologist. *Am J Orthod Dentofacial Orthop* 2011;139:10, 12, 14, 16.

Steed PA & Wexler GB (2001). Temporomandibular disorders-traumatic etiology *vs.* nontraumatic etiology: a clinical and methodological inquiry into symptomatology and treatment outcomes. *J Craniomandib Pract* 2001;19:188-194.

Türp JC, Greene CS, Strub JR (2008). Dental occlusion: a critical reflection on past, present and future concepts. *J Oral Rehabil* 2008;35:446-453

Wänman A (1987). Craniomandibular disorders in adolescents. A longitudinal study in an urban Swedish population. *Swed Dent J* 1987; Suppl:44:1-61.

Zarb GA & Thompson GW (1975). The treatment of patients with temporomandibular joint pain dysfunction syndrome. *J Canad Dent Assn* 1975;7:410-417.

Send Orders for Reprints to reprints@benthamscience.net

CHAPTER 3

Occlusion and Temporomandibular Disorders

Abstract: The relation between retruded contact position (RCP), oblique slide from RCP to intercuspal position (ICP), and temporomandibular disorders (TMDs) has not been demonstrated. Recently, occlusal discrepancy between habitual occlusal position (HOP) and bite plate-induced occlusal position (BPOP) has been reported to be related with sign (TMJ clicking) of TMD in a cross-sectional study. And elimination of the occlusal discrepancy is inferred to cure TMDs.

Keywords: Retruded contact position, intercuspal position, occlusion, conservative treatment, occlusal adjustment, terminal hinge closure, counseling, clinical dysfunction index, placebo treatment, occlusal splint, comprehensive treatment, malocclusion, intra-articular injection, randomized controlled trial, bite plate-induced occlusal position, habitual occlusal position.

1. TERMINOLOGY

CR (centric relation) is defined as follows: 1. The maxillomandibular relationship in which the condyles articulate with the thinnest avascular portion of their respective disks with the complex in the anterior-superior position against the shapes of the eminencies. This position is independent of tooth contact. This position is clinically discernible when the mandible is directed superior and anteriorly. It is restricted to a purely rotary movement about the transverse horizontal axis (GPT-5) (The Academy of Prosthodontics, 1999). RCP (retruded contact position): that guided occlusal relationship occurring at the most retruded position of the condyles in the joint cavities. A position that may be more retruded than the centric relation position (The Academy of Prosthodontics, 1999). ICP (intercuspal position): maximal intercuspal position. The complete intercuspation of the opposing teeth independent of condylar position, sometimes referred to as the best fit of the teeth regardless of the condylar position-called also maximal intercuspation (The Academy of Prosthodontics, 1999). HOP (habitual occlusal position) is defined by Torii and Chiwata as follows: This mandibular position is obtained by voluntary jaw closing while in an upright position and regarded as mandibular position induced by the jow motor program of the central nervous sytem (Torii K & Chiwata I, 2005). BPOP (bite plate induced induced occlusal position): This mandibular position is obtained during voluntary jaw closing, while in an upright position and after wearing an anterior bite plate for a short period of time and regarded as muscular contact position, induced by altering the motor program (Torii K & Chiwata I, 2005).

2. INTRODUCTION

Many studies of occlusal adjustment have been performed to demonstrate the effectiveness on TMDs and a cause-and-effect relation between occlusion and TMDs. In addition, the studies regarding the effects on the stomatognathic system with artificial interferences have been performed. However, clear occlusal factors have not been found. Therefore, conservative treatment modalities (appliance therapy, physical medicine medication, *etc.*) are the main treatments at present. However, these treatments are symptomatic and the recurrence will inevitably occur. TMDs are not fatal diseases but influence the quality of life (headache, tinnitus, painful tongue, *etc.*). Therefore, we have to find out the causes of TMDs and establish the treatment for it. It is clear that occlusion has great influence on the stomatognathic system, and probably the causes of TMDs exist in occlusion.

3. OCCLUSAL ADJUSTMENT

The occlusal adjustment performed in Europe since 1970s was mainly based on the concept proposed by Krough-Poulsen and Olsson (Krough-Poulsen WG & Olsson A, 1966). The occlusal adjustment was performed to eliminate unilateral premature contacts in the retruded contact position (RCP) and interferences between RCP and intercuspal position (ICP) causing lateral displacement of the mandible. The RCP was located by passively guiding of the mandible to the first tooth contact in the terminal hinge closure. Tsukiyama *et al.* reviewed the published experimental studies on occlusal adjustments and TMDs, and concluded that the experimental evidence reviewed was neither convincing nor powerful enough to support the performance of occlusal therapy as a general method for treating a nonacute temporomandibular disorder, bruxism, or headache (Tsukiyama *et al.*, 2001). Kopp performed short term evaluation of counseling and occlusal adjustment in patients with TMDs, and reported that the score of subjective dysfunction was reduced significantly and clinical dysfunction score was reduced significantly. Further, Kopp concluded that counseling may reduce the subjective symptoms; and occlusal adjustment may reduce the clinical signs of mandibular dysfunction involving the TMJ, but that the individual variation in response is substantial. Kopp described as follows: the agreement between changes of the subjective and the clinical dysfunction scores following the occlusal adjustment was poor. Changes in the subjective dysfunction score were often associated with corresponding changes in the clinical dysfunction score, but not the reverse. An explanation to this finding could be that changes in the clinical dysfunction score, even considerable ones, are not necessarily perceived by the patients as significant changes of their condition. The subjective response to changes in the clinical dysfunction index is also likely to be different for the different variables included. The perception and interpretation of pain, which is a major part in the subjective experience of mandibular dysfunction, are strongly influenced by psychological factors and personal characteristics. The poor agreement previously found between pain in the masticatory system and palpatory tenderness of the masticatory muscles and the high frequency of palpatory findings, which could be found in persons without pain also reflect the discrepancy between subjective and clinical dysfunction. It seems that the clinical dysfunction index is sensitive for even minor alterations in the clinical conditions and that such a score should be used in combination with the patient's subjective evaluation in future clinical treatment trials (Kopp S, 1979). Forssell *et al.* performed a double-blind study on the effect of occlusal adjustment on TMDs in which 48 patients in the treatment group received occlusal adjustment and 19 of them received splint therapy, and in the placebo group all 43 patients received mock adjustment. They reported that placebo treatment and real treatment were equally effective in relieving symptoms of TMDs, but there was significantly more reduction in signs of TMDs in the real treatment group than in the placebo group. And they concluded that the elimination of occlusal disturbances was an effective treatment for TMDs. They also described that the elimination of occlusal disturbances was the effective treatment because the changes in clinical signs of mandibular dysfunction were independent of the use of splints as an aid to the treatment. On the other hand, the effect achieved with occlusal adjustment as compared with placebo treatment in the present study clearly disputes the argument that all kinds of treatment, including placebo, are equally effective in the treatment of mandibular dysfunction (Forssell H *et al.*, 1986). Forssell *et al.* also reported the similar results, and described that the results are complementary to our earlier clinical studies and corroborate the conclusion that improvements after occlusal adjustment exceed those after placebo treatment (Forssell H *et al.*, 1987). Wenneberg *et al.* compared occlusal adjustment and other stomatognathic treatment. In their study patients were randomly divided into two treatment groups of 15 patients each, and one group was prescribed occlusal equilibration according to the Panky-Mann-Schuyler method and the other group received various kinds of stomatognathic therapies (maxillary full-coverage acrylic resin occlusal splint, mandibular exercises and minor occlusal adjustment of less than 5 minutes duration). They reported that the clinical dysfunction score used was significantly diminished only in the splint therapy group. And they further described that a combined treatment regimen, including an occlusal splint, was more effective than occlusal adjustment alone, especially with regard to clinical signs of dysfunction. And more visits were needed for the extensive occlusal adjustment performed than for the other type of therapy, and a stable occlusion was obtained and perceived as such by most patients as increased occlusal comfort. However, a disadvantage was that six patients (40%) complained of increased thermal sensitivity after the equilibration. It is sometimes suggested that if success in treatment is not achieved, then the adjustment has not been done properly or has not reached the ultimate goal of "occlusal stability". However, there is no scientific support for this concept. On the contrary, today there is more evidence suggesting that occlusion, including "occlusal stability", plays a minor etiologic role in TMDs. Therefore, continuing occlusal adjustment after elimination of obvious, marked interferences that may disturb occlusal function is neither cost effective nor scientifically supported. Such an adjustment can usually be performed within half an hour in most patients and may be considered a useful method for the treatment of some functional disturbances of masticatory system (Wenneberg B *et al.*, 1988). On the other hand, Kirveskari *et al.* performed prophylactically occlusal adjustment for non-symptomatic dental students and described that prophylactic occlusal adjustment appears to be effective in reducing occurrence of symptoms of TMDs, and possibly also the occurrence of clinical signs (Kirveskari P *et al.*, 1989). Vallon *et al.* evaluated the short-term effect of occlusal adjustment on TMDs and described that occlusal adjustment provides a general subjective improvement of TMDs. They also described that occlusal adjustment did not influence the clinical signs of TMD in this study. An explanation might be that the clinical variables registered are not sensitive or specific enough to show changes induced by treatment, as indicated by the subjective response, or the observation time may have been too short. The initial degree of clinical dysfunction was low, according to the clinical dysfunction score in both groups, corresponding to the index value of I, which may indicate a too low sensitivity of the index for this purpose. The short-term effect of the occlusal adjustment on subjective symptoms of TMD has generally reported to be good. However, it should be noted that there is often a discrepancy between clinical signs and subjective symptoms and that signs of TMDs are commoner than subjective symptoms in the population. The need for treatment is mainly determined by the severity of the experienced symptoms, and evaluation of treatment effect should therefore be based at least partly on the effect on these symptoms. If the patient's evaluation of symptoms is taken as a measurement, occlusal adjustment is a treatment alternative for TMDs (Vallon D *et al.*, 1991). Vallon *et al.* also described that occlusal adjustment is a treatment modality with a statistically significant short-term effect on symptoms of TMDs of muscular origin and superior to counseling (Vallon D *et al.*, 1995). In addition, Vallon and Nilner performed two-year follow-up of the effect of occlusal adjustment and reported that 48% patients in the treatment group and 84% in the control group had demanded rescue treatment. Eleven patients in the treatment group and 3 patients in the control group without rescue treatment, reported overall subjective improvement. No difference was found between the groups regarding overall intensity of pain expressed by the visual analog scale. When all kinds of treatment were taken into account, 70% and 79% of the patients in the treatment group and control group reported overall subjective improvement at follow-up. Further, they concluded that the majority of the patients with TMDs required a comprehensive treatment program (Vallon D & Nilner M, 1997). Karppinen *et al.* compared occlusal adjustment and mock-adjustment for patients suffering from chronic cervicobrachial pain and/or headache, and reported that in the long-term, the response was better in the patients who had undergone occlusal adjustment than in the mock-adjustment. It is further described as follows: The NIH (National Institute of Health, U.S.A.) Technology Assessment Conference Statement (1996) advises against the use of occlusal therapy for TMDs. However, the controversy over the role of occlusion in TMDs continues. In the present study, occlusal adjustment proved effective in the treatment of chronic neck and shoulder pain, and/or chronic headache. It seems warranted to bring attention to the possibility that faulty dental occlusion in part explains why the response to physical therapy of chronic neck/shoulder pain may not be always good in the long term (Karppinen K *et al.*, 1999). In contrast with these studies mentioned above, Tsolka *et al.* clinically evaluated occlusal adjustment by a double-blind method, and reported that there was no significant difference in the improvements on the signs and symptoms obtained by real or mock adjustment (Tsolka P *et al.*, 1992). Kirveskari described as follows: Controlled clinical trials have yielded results that are difficult to explain unless occlusal factors have a causal role in temporomandibular disorders. Controlled clinical trials also suggest an effect for occlusal adjustment on chronic headaches and on chronic neck and shoulder pain in comparison with conventional treatments. In view of the possibility that occlusal factors have a causal role in temporomandibular disorders, research efforts on the role of occlusion should be intensified, and teaching should be revised accordingly (Kirveskari P, 1997). In addition, Kirveskari and Jämsä currently described that systemic elimination of occlusal interferences significantly reduced the incidence of requests for the treatment of symptoms in the head and cervicobrachial region. This is in contrast the view that there is no, or at best, an insignificant health risk from occlusal interferences (Kirveskari P & Jämsä T, 2009).

4. OCCLUSAL FACTORS IN CLINICAL STUDIES

Mohlin and Kopp examined 56 patients with TMDs and recorded three types of occlusal interferences: premature contact in RCP, interferences between RCP and ICP causing a lateral slide of the mandible ≥ 0.5 mm, and mediotrusion interferences (cuspal contacts on the nonworking side that prevent contact on the working side in lateral movement). They reported that no correlation was found between any of the interferences or malocclusion and the severity of mandibular pain and dysfunction as judged by the dysfunction index. They described as follows: When the clinical dysfunction index was used, none of the occlusal interferences or malocclusions could be related to the degree of pain and dysfunction as judged from the multiple tests. This means that patients with any of these interferences or malocclusions do not differ from those without with respect to severity of pain and dysfunction. This finding indicates that there are other important factors in the etiology of mandibular pain and dysfunction than occlusal factors. Mediotrusion interferences were more frequent among individuals with tipped teeth and bilateral cross bite. RP-IP interferences were more frequent in individuals than in those without uni- or bilateral cross bite. The present results therefore indicate that tipping of teeth and bilateral cross bite involve a risk of mediotrusion interferences and that uni- and bilateral cross bite involves a risk of RP-IP interferences. There are still many questions to be answered in this field. First of all, we are still in doubt about the importance of above-mentioned interferences. This is important when considering the indications for the treatment of tipped teeth and cross bite. That forced cross bite (unilateral) can cause a disturbed muscular pattern has been shown earlier. Their finding that bilateral cross bite more than the unilateral type could be related to certain interferences needs to be further examined. They described that the possible influence on pain and dysfunction of a frontal open bite can be explained in several ways. One possibility is that the number of tooth contacts is decreased, thereby creating an unstable occlusion. Another is that there could be a different pattern of muscular activity in patients with open bite. We know that the activity in the masticatory muscles varies with the morphology of the facial skeleton, so that individuals with parallelism between the jawbases and between the mandibular occlusal plane and the mandibular line show greater muscular activity, especially during chewing and maximal bite. Because of this, there is a need to make a distinction between skeletal and pure dento-alveolar open bite in future studies (Mohlin B & Kopp S, 1978). Kopp and Wenneberg evaluated the long-term effect (2 year) of occlusal treatment (including occlusal splint therapy and occlusal adjustment) and intra-articular injections of a mixture of corticosteroid and local anesthetic in two groups of patients with pain and dysfunction in the TMJ. They reported as follows: Both sorts of treatment reduced the subjective symptoms and the clinical signs significantly, but the reduction was significantly greater after the intra-articular injections. The effect of the injections was less efficient in patients with radiographic signs of remodeling of the TMJ and general joint symptoms. It was concluded that both intra-articular injections of corticosteroid combined with local anesthetic and occlusal treatment have a long term palliative effect on TMJ pain and dysfunction. The intra-articular treatment, however, had a greater effect on the clinical signs (Kopp S & Wenneberg B, 1981). On the other hand, De Laat *et al.* investigated correlation between occlusal and articular parameters and symptoms of TMJ dysfunction in the group of 121 final-year dental students, and reported that an asymmetric slide from RCP to ICP correlated with pain in the TMJ during palpation, and they concluded that although several significant correlations exist between occlusal parameters and signs and symptoms of TMJ dysfunction in the present study, the occlusal relationships alone cannot possibly be responsible for etiology of TMJ dysfunction. This tends to support the multifactorial etiology claimed in previous studies. The examination of the selected set of occlusal factors does not appear to have a predictive value in determining whether a patient will show a particular sign or symptom (De Laat A *et al.*, 1986). Egermark-Eriksson *et al.* described from the result of their longitudinal study as follows: TMJ sounds positively correlated with lateral deviation of the mandible between RCP and ICP in all age groups, and an attempt to analyze the longitudinal relationship of occlusal interference with signs and symptoms of mandibular dysfunction did not reveal any strong correlations. Therefore, the results are interpreted as supporting the heterogeneous and multifactorial nature of functional disturbances of the masticatory system (Egermark-Eriksson I *et al.*, 1987). Seligman *et al.* examined dental attrition in young adults, and reported that dental attrition was not associated with the presence or absence of TMJ clicking, TMJ tenderness, or masticatory muscle tenderness (Seligman DA *et al.*, 1988). Seligman and Pullinger also reported that asymmetric RCP-ICP slides were more prevalent in women with reducing disk displacement and large RCP-ICP slides, asymmetric slides, and anterior open bite were associated with osteoarthrosis, but this study could not state if these associations were etiologic or secondary, and they described as follows: Belief in the contribution of occlusion to the etiology of craniomandibular pain and dysfunction, together with the dental and mandibular orthopedic treatments of these disorders, keeps this field of medicine within dental practice. Notwithstanding, contemporary research has been unable to support a strong occlusomorphological linkage to craniomandibular disorders. It has been said that dento-occlusal factors are not strongly correlated to treatment outcome, are not good predictors of dysfunction, and are not reliable for predicting symptom severity. It may be that a malocclusion must be present for a considerable time period to induce an effect. The multifactorial etiology and pathophysiology of craniomandibular disorders are well accepted today, and occlusion may be only one feature of this mechanism. Biophysiology would expect some contribution of morphology to functional status. The inability of much past research to find a consensus on morpho-occlusal associations may be the result of poorly defined experimental and control groups. In addition, many prior studies circularly defined the study population according to the symptom being tested. We believe the importance of studying discrete diagnostic groups and comparing them to uncompromised control populations cannot be overemphasized. This study has demonstrated several significant relationships that clarify some of the past conflicts. By studying well-defined patient diagnostic groups rather than symptoms and comparing the patient groups to a control group, selective aspects of occlusion have been shown to be more closely associated with TMJ disorders than indicated in many past studies with less specified populations. It is important to emphasize that epidemiologic studies, while demonstrating associations, cannot prove the etiologic contributions of occlusion. Some occlusal features may be the consequence of articular disorders, some may encourage disorders and their progression, and others may be protective (Seligman DA & Pullinger AG, 1989). McNamara *et al.* described that signs and symptoms of TMD occur in healthy individuals and increase with age, particularly during adolescence; thus, TM disorders that originate during various types of dental treatment may not be related to the treatment but may be a naturally occurring phenomenon (McNamara JA *et al.*, 1995). This description is in agreement with the results of Torii's longitudinal study in which persistent clicking in the TMJ began at 11 or 12 years of age once the permanent dentition had been achieved and the clicking did not relate to dental treatment, but significantly smaller bite force (Torii K, 2011). McNamara *et al.* summarized as follows: The multiple factor analysis of Pullinger and colleagues has indicated that there is a relatively low association of occlusal factors in characterizing TMD. This association, however, is not zero, and several occlusal features characterized the diagnostic groups: 1) Skeletal anterior open bite; 2) Overjet greater than 6 to 7 mm; 3) RCP/ICP slides greater than 4 mm; Unilateral lingual cross bite; 5) Five or more missing posterior teeth. The first three factors often are associated with TMJ arthropathies and may be the result of an osseous or ligamentous change within the temporomandibular articulation. Overall, Seligman estimates that the total contribution of occlusal factors to the multifactorial characterization of TMD patients is about 10% to 20 %, with other factors, both pronounced and subtle, interacting and providing the remaining 80% to 90% of the differences between patients and healthy subjects. Regarding the relationship of orthodontic treatment to TMD, they summarized as follows: 1) Signs and symptoms of TMD occur in healthy individuals. 2) Signs and symptoms of TMD increase with age, particularly during adolescence. Thus, TMD that originates during treatment may not be related to the treatment. 3) Orthodontic treatment performed during adolescence generally does not increase or decrease the odds of developing TMD later in life. 4) The extraction of teeth as part of an orthodontic treatment plan does not increase the risk of TMD. 5) There is no elevated risk for TMD associated with any particular type of orthodontic mechanics. 6) Although a stable occlusion is a reasonable orthodontic treatment goal, not achieving a specific gnathologic ideal occlusion does not result in TMD signs and symptoms. 7) No method of TMJ disorder prevention has been demonstrated. 8) When more severe TMD signs and symptoms are present, simple treatments can alleviate them in most patients. Thus, according to the existing literature, the relationship of TMD to occlusion and orthodontic treatment is minor. The important question that still remains in dentistry is how this minor contribution can be identified within the population of TMD patients. Future research should be directed towards developing a more complete understanding of these occlusal factors so that reliable criteria can be developed to assist the dental practitioner in deciding when dental therapy plays a role in the management of TM disorders. Reliable criteria likely would spare many TMD patients significant dental therapies and related health costs. Until such criteria are developed, the dental profession should be encouraged to manage TMD symptoms with reversible therapies, only considering permanent alterations of the occlusion in patients with very unique circumstances (McNamara JA *et al*. 1995). Forssell *et al*. performed a systemic review of randomized controlled trials (RCTs) of occlusal treatment studies and summarized as follows: *Splint therapy* was found superior to three control treatments (ultrasound, palliative treatment and palatal splint) and comparable to twelve control treatments. *Occlusal adjustment* was found to be equal to control treatment in two studies and inferior to control treatment in one. On the basis of our analysis we conclude that RCTs seem to suggest that the use of occlusal splints may be beneficial in the treatment of TMD, but the evidence is scarce. On the other hand, there is no evidence for the use of occlusal adjustment. The small number and also the poor quality of most of the RCTs analyzing occlusal adjustment do not, however, allow any definite conclusions. In addition, it is described as follows: The debate about occlusal treatments in TMD has a long history and does not seem to be calming down. What became obvious from this systemic review was the small number of randomized controlled trials. It was shocking to realize that we are so short of good studies in this vigorously debated field. The present systemic review on occlusal treatments in TMD could not reach any firm conclusions, but we hope to have highlighted the areas of importance to be considered when planning future studies. There is an obvious need for well designed controlled studies to analyze the current clinical practices. The existence of some high quality RCTs enhances our confidence in the ability of the researchers to be able to establish a clear scientific basis for the treatment of TMD (Forssell H *et al.*, 1999; Forssell H & Kalso E, 2004).

5. EXPERIMENTAL OCCLUSAL INTERFERENCE

Riise and Sheikholeslam inserted an artificial occlusal interference on the maxillary right first molar (the medial facet of the disto-buccal cusp) and observed the electrical activity of the anterior temporal and masseter muscles. They reported that after 48 hours there was a significant increase of the activity in the anterior temporal muscles and the increased activity persisted until the interference was removed, and described that in the long run, the hyperactivity may be followed by structural adaptation such as teeth movements, muscular reactions and remodeling of the TMJ or may lead to pathological changes in the masticatory system, and they concluded that the present results indicate that there is postural activity in the anterior temporal and sometimes in the masseter muscles, and that experimental occlusal interferences similar to those often produced in the daily dental practice of occlusal rehabilitation, such as fillings, crowns, and bridges affect the neuromuscular pattern of postural activity in the mandibular elevators at rest. The results may not be valid for all types of interferences (Riise C & Sheikholeslam A, 1982). Magnusson and Enbom performed a study of experimental balancing-side interferences in two groups of young, healthy women without signs or symptoms of TMDs. Each group contained 12 individuals. In one of the groups, balancing-side interferences were applied bilaterally, whereas the application was simulated in the other group. Ten individuals in the experimental group reported one or more subjective symptoms during the 2-weeks, whereas seven exhibited clinical signs of dysfunction. The most common symptom was headache, and the most common clinical sign was muscle tender to palpation. In the control group, three individuals reported subjective symptoms, and three had clinical signs of dysfunction. One week after elimination of the interferences, all signs and symptoms had disappeared in all individuals but two. In these two subjects, it took 6 weeks before pre-experimental conditions were restored. Magnusson and Enbom concluded that there is no simple relationship between interferences and signs and symptoms of dysfunction and how the individual reacts to local factors depends on his or her psychic condition (Magnusson T & Enbom L, 1984). Belser and Hannam investigated the influence of artificially altered working-side occlusal guidance on masticatory muscles and jaw movement, and summarized as follows: The effect of four different occlusal situations (group function, canine guidance, working side occlusal interference, and hyperbalancing occlusal interference) on electromyographic (EMG) activity in jaw elevator muscles and related mandibular movement was investigated in 12 subjects. When a naturally acquired group function was temporarily and artificially changed into a dominant canine guidance, significant general reduction of elevator muscle activity was observed when subjects exerted full isometric tooth-clenching efforts in a lateral mandibular position. The original muscular coordination pattern (relative contraction from muscle to muscle) remained unaltered during this test. With respect to unilateral chewing, no significant alterations in the activity or coordination of the muscles occurred when an artificial canine guidance was introduced. Introduction of a hyper balancing occlusal contact caused significant alterations in muscle activity and coordination during maximal tooth clenching in a lateral mandibular position. A marked shift of temporal muscle EMG activity toward the side of the interference and unchanged bilateral activity of the two masseter muscles were observed. The results suggest that canine-protected occlusions do not significantly alter muscle activity during mastication but significantly reduce muscle activity during parafunctional clenching. They also suggest that non-working side contacts dramatically alter the distribution of muscle activity during parafunctional clenching, and that this redistribution may affect the nature of reaction forces at the temporomandibular joints (Belser UC & Hannam AG, 1985).

6. CONTROVERSY REGARDING OCCLUSION AND TMDs

The NIH (National Institutes of Health) /NIDR (National Institute of Dental Research), Technology Conference on Management of Temporomandibular disorders held in May 1996 in the USA concluded that there is no data to support many commonly held beliefs in TMD, nor is there data to support the superiority of any method of management as being better than a placebo. It stated that occlusal adjustments are invasive and that superiority of such treatment over other non-invasive therapies has not been demonstrated in randomized controlled prospective trials and these conclusions were justified by the literature which described the proceedings (National Institutes of Health Technology Assessment Conference on Management of Temporomandibular Disorders. Bethesta, Md., April 29- May 1, 1996., 1997). In addition, Greene *et al.* stated that it is strongly recommended that, unless there are specific and justifiable indications to the contrary, treatment should be based on the use of conservative and reversible therapeutic modalities (Greene CS *et al.*, 1998). On the other hand, Dawson strongly contradicted these statements (Dawson PE, 1999). The conclusions of the panel seemed to be too early, because the relation between occlusion and TMDs has not thoroughly been investigated at present.

7. CURRENTLY OBTAINED EVIDENCE OF OCCLUSAL FACTOR

Torii and Chiwata compared habitual occlusal position (HOP) and bite plate-induced occlusal position (BPOP) in volunteers with and without TMJ sounds (Torii K & Chiwata I, 2005). While recording the HOP, a vinyl polysiloxane bite registration material was applied with syringe over the occlusal surfaces and then subject was asked to close into maximum intercuspation, and hold that position until the material was set (approximately one minute). To standardize the BPOP recording method, the subject was conditioned neuromuscularly with an anterior flat bite plate, against which he or she tapped and slid the lower anterior teeth for five minutes. After conditioning, the plate was removed, and a registration material was applied over the occlusal surfaces, and the subject was asked to close his or her mouth. Three interocclusal records were obtained for each occlusal position. The trimmed interocclusal record was interposed between the casts mounted on a three-dimensionally analyzing apparatus modified from an articulator, and then the positions were marked using needles (Fig. **1a**).

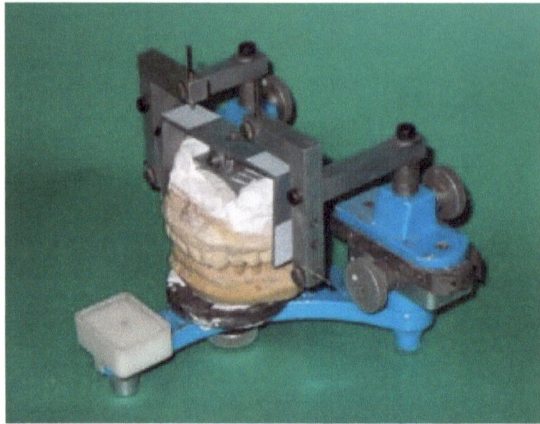

Figure 1a: Three-dimensionally recording apparatus.

The recording frame is attached to the upper cast. Mandibular positions are recorded on the frame on both sides using needles.

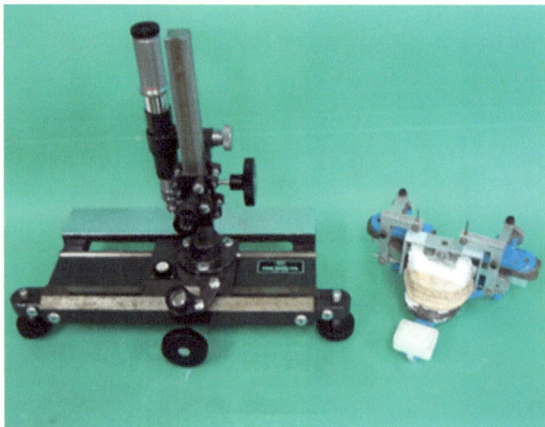

Figure 1b: Measuring microscope.

All registrations were read using a measuring microscope with resolution of 0.01 mm (Fig. **1b**).

The results are following: The mean variations on all axes and standard deviations are shown in Fig. **2**;

In the control group, no significant differences in variations were observed between the HOP and the BPOP for all axes($p>0.2$); In the group of subjects with TMJ sounds, while no significant differences in variations were observed between the HOP and the BPOP for the x- (mediolateral) and y- (anteroposterior) ($p>0.2$), the difference for the z- (superioinferior) was significant ($p<0.01$); While no significant differences in BPOP variations were observed between the groups of the subjects with TMJ sounds and controls for the y- and z-axes ($p>0.05$), the difference for the x-axis was significant ($p<0.05$); The mean difference between the HOP and BPOP is shown in Fig. **3**; The standard deviations of the mean difference between the HOP and BPOP in control subjects were ±0.12 mm on the

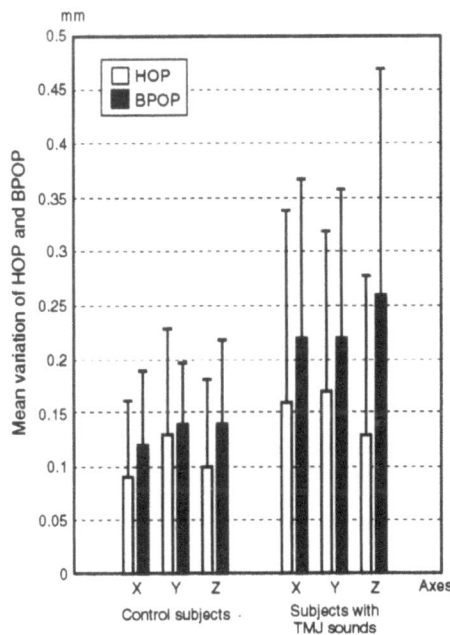

Figure 2: Mean variations of HOP and BPOP on each axis for subjects with TMJ sounds and for control subjects.

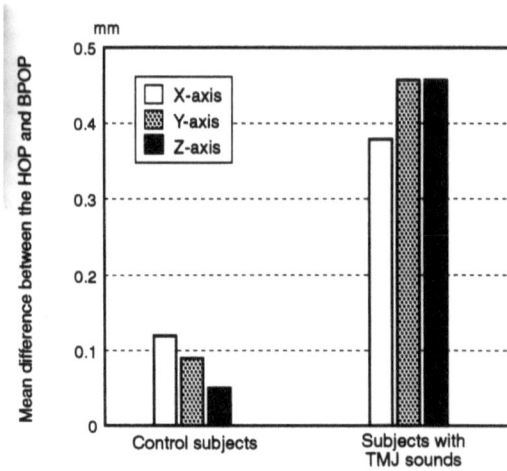

Figure 3: Mean differences between HOP and BPOP on each axis for subjects with TMJ sounds and for control subjects.

x-axis, ±0.07 mm, on the y-axis and ±0.06 mm on the z-axis, whereas those in subjects with TMJ on the y-axis and ±0.06 mm on the z-axis, whereas those in subjects with TMJ sounds were ±0.37 mm on the x-axis, ±0.33 mm on the y-axis and ±0.64 mm on the z-axis; The mean differences between both groups were significant on all axes ($p<0.05$); The statistical differences between the HOP and BPOP in each subject were significantly associated with subjects having TMJ sounds (Table **1**).

Table 1: Statistical differences between HOP-BPOP and TMJ sounds

Table 1 Statistical Differences Between HOP-BPOP and TMJ Sounds		
Statistical difference between HOP and BPOP	Subjects w/TMJ sounds	Control subjects
No difference	1	13
Difference	14	2

HOP: habitual occlusal position
BPOP: bite plane induced occlusal position
(The relationship between the statistical difference of HOP-BPOP and TMJ sounds was significant ($p=0.000007$, using Fisher's exact test.)

Mohl stated that the muscular contact position is usually consistent with ICP in asymptomatic subjects sitting with the head in an upright position (Mohl ND, 1991). Brill *et al.* postulated that the coincidence of MP (muscular contact position) and ICP constitutes a physiological condition: where the two positions do not coincide, a pathological or potentially pathological condition is likely to be present (Brill N *et al.*, 1959). Moyers described that the continued presence of occlusal disharmony in centric position might cause a new reflex pattern of pathways to be repeatedly used, causing the new position of the mandible to resemble ICP. In such case, a discrepancy between ICP and centric relation might emerge (Moyers RE, 1956). It is thought that the occlusal discrepancy between the HOP and BPOP might emerge with occlusal interferences in physiologically muscular closure. Therefore, eliminating the interferences in the BPOP might make the HOP coincide with the BPOP. In order to demonstrate the causal factor of the occlusal discrepancy between the HOP and BPOP, it is essential that the artificially induced occlusal discrepancy causes TMD. However, artificially inducing the occlusal discrepancy seems to be difficult, because the discrepancy is thought to emerge during long term of the mixed dentition (Torii K, 2011).

SUMMARY

Although it has not been demonstrated that the occlusal discrepancy between HOP and BPOP inevitably causes TMD, the occlusal examination should be performed for a patient with TMD about whether the discrepancy exists or not.

REFERENCES

Belser UC & Hannam AG (1985). The influence of altered working-side occlusal guidance on masticatory muscle and related jaw movement. *J Prosthet Dent* 1985;53:406-413.

Brill N, Lammie GA, Osborne J, Perry HT (1959). Madibular positions and mandibular movements. *Brit Dent J* 1959;106:391-400.

Dawson PE (1999). Position paper regarding diagnosis, management, and treatment of temporomandibular disorders. *J Prosthet Dent* 1999;81:174-178.

De Laat A, van Steenberghe D, Lesaffre E (1986). Occlusal relationships and temporomandibular joint dysfunction. Pat II: Correlations between occlusal and articular parameters and symptoms of TMJ dysfunction by means of stepwise logistic regression. *J Prosthet Dent* 1986;55:116-121.

Egermark-Eriksson I, Carlsson GE, Magnusson T (1987). A long-term epidemiological study of the relationship between occlusal factors and mandibular dysfunction in children and adolescents. *J Dent Res* 1987;66:67-71.

Forssell H, Kirveskari P, Kangasniemi P (1986). Effect of occlusal adjustment on mandibular dysfunction. A double-blind study. *Acta Odontol Scand* 1986;44:63-69.

Forssell H, Kirveskari P, Kangasniemi P (1987). Response to occlusal treatment in headache patients previously treated by mock occlusal adjustment. *Acta Odontol Scand* 1987;45:77-80.

Forssell H, Kalso E, Koskela P, Vehmanen R, Puuka P, Alanen P (1999). Occlusal treatment in temporomandibualr disorders: a qualitative systemic review of randomized controlled trials. *Pain* 1999;83:549-560.

Forssell H, Kalso E (2004). Application of principle of evidence-based medicine to occlusal treatment for temporomandibular disorders: Are there lessons to be learned? *J Orofac Pain* 2004;18:9-22.

Greene CS, Mohl ND, McNeill C, Clark GT, Truelove EL (1998). Temporomandibular disorders and science: A response to the critics. *J Prosthet Dent* 1998;80:214-215.

Karppinen K, Eklund S, Suoninen E, Eskelin M, Kirveskari P (1999). Adjustment of dental occlusion in treatment of chronic cervicobrachial pain and headache. *J Oral Rehabil* 1999;26:715-721.

Kirveskari P, Le Bell Y, Salonen M, Forssell H (1989). Effect of elimination of occlusal interferences on signs and symptoms of craniomandibular disorder in young adults. *J Oral Rehabil* 1989;16:21-26.

Kirveskari P (1997). The role of occlusal adjustment in the management of temporomandibular disorders. *Oral Surg Oral Med Oral Pathol Oral Radiol Endod* 1997;83:87-90.

Kirveskari P & Jämsä T (2009). Health risk from occlusalinterferences in females. *Eur J Orthod* 2009;31:490-495.

Kopp S (1979). Short term evaluation of counseling and occlusal adjustment in patients with mandibular dysfunction involving the temporomandibular joint. *J Oral Rehabil* 1979;6:101-109.

Kopp S & Wenneberg B (1981). Effects of occlusal treatment and intra-articular injections on temporomandibular joint pain and dysfunction. *Acta Odontol Scand* 1981;39:87-96.

Krogh-Poulsen W & Olsson A (1966). Occlusal disharmonies and dysfunction of the stomatognathic system. *Dent Clin North Am* 1966;Nov.:627-635.

Magnusson T & Enbom L (1984). Signs and symptoms of mandibular dysfunction after introduction of experimental balancing-side interferences. *Acta Odontol Scand* 1984;42:129-135.

McNamara JA, Seligman DA, Okeson JP (1995). Occlusion, orthodontic treatment, and temporomandibular disorders: A review. *J Orofac Pain*1995;9:73-90.

Mohl ND (1991): Introduction to occlusion. In: Mohl ND, Zarb GA, Carlsson GE, Rugh JD, ed. *A textbook of occlusion.* Chicago: Quintessence, 1991:15-23.

Mohlin B & Kopp S (1978). A clinical study on the relationship between malocclusions, occlusal interferences and mandibular pain and dysfunction. *Swed Dent J* 1978;2:105-112.

Moyers RE (1956). Some physiologic considerations of centric and other jaw relations. *J Prosthet Dent* 1956;6:183-194.

National Institutes of Health Assessment on Management of Temporomandibular Disorders. Bethesda, Md., April 29- May 1, 1996. Oral Surge Oral Med Oral Pathol Oral Radiol Endod 1997;83:49-50.

Riise C & Sheikholeslam A (1982). The influence of experimental interfering occlusal contacts on the postural ativity of the anterior temporal and masseter muscles in youg adults. *J Oral Rehabil* 1982;9:419-425.

Seligman DA, Pullinger AG, Solberg WK (1988). The prevalence of dental attrition and its association with factors of age, gender, occlusion, and TMJ symptomatology. *J Dent Res* 1988;67:1323-1333.

Seligman DA & Pullinger AG (1989). Association of occlusal variables among refined TM patient diagnostic groups. *J Craniomandib Disord Facial Oral Pain* 1989;3:227-236.

The Academy of Prosthodontics (1999). *Glossary of Prosthodontic Terms.* 7-th ed. St. Louis: C.V. Mosby Co., 1999.

Tsukiyama Y, Baba K, Clark GT (2001). An evidence-based assessment of occlusal adjustment as a treatmentfor temporomandibular disorders. *J Prosthet Dent* 2001;86:57-66.

Torii K & Chiwata I (2005). Relationship between habitual occlusal position and flat bite plane induced occlusal position in volunteers with and without temporomandibular joint sounds. *J Craniomandib Pract* 2005;23:16-21.

Torii K (2011). Longitudinal course of temporomandibular joint sounds in Japanese children and adolescents. *Head & Face Medicine* 2011, 7:17., Available from http://www.head-face-med.com/content/7/1/17

Tsolka P, Morris RW, Preiskel HW (1992). Occlusal adjustment therapy for craniomandibular disorders: A clinical assessment by a double-blind method. *J Prosthet Dent* 1992;68:957-964.

Vallon D, Ekberg EC, Nilner M, Kopp S (1991). Sort-term effect of occlusal adjustment on craniomandibular disorders including headaches. *Acta Odontol Scand* 1991;49:89-96.

Vallon D, Ekberg EC, Nilner M, Kopp S (1995). Occlusal adjustment in patients with craniomandibular disorders including headaches. A 3- and 6-month follow-up. *Acta Odontol Scand* 1995;53:55-59.

Vallon D & Nilner M (1997). A longitudinal follow-up of the effect of occlusal adjustment in patients with craniomandibular disorders. *Swed Dent J* 1997;21:85-91.

Wenneberg B, Nystrom T, Carlsson GE (1988). Occlusal equilibration and other stomatognathic treatment in patients with mandibular dysfunction and headache. *J Prosthet Dent* 1988;59:478-489.

CHAPTER 4

Reference Position for Occlusal Analysis and Equilibration

Abstract: The value of retruded contact position (RCP) as a reference position for an occlusal analysis has not been demonstrated. On the other hand, muscular contact position (MCP) has been found to be important for a reference position in occlusal analysis and occlusal equilibration.

Keywords: Reference position, muscular contact position, occlusal equilibration, retruded contact position, intercuspal position, occlusal analysis, Gothic arch tracing, terminal hinge movement, muscular position, Chin-point guidance, habitual closure, double-blind method, ligamentous position, tooth position, postural reflex, centric relation, gnathosonic technique, occlusal splint, median occlusion, electromyographic silent period, Myocentric, bite plate-induced occlusal position.

1. TERMINOLOGY

RCP (retruded contact position) is defined as guided occlusal relationship occurring at the most retruded position of the condyles in the joint cavities. A position that may be more retruded than the centric relation position (The Academy of Prosthodontics, 1999). ICP (intercuspal position): maximal intercuspal position, the complete intercuspation of the opposing teeth independent of condylar position, sometimes referred to as the best fit of the teeth regardless of the condylar position-called also maximal intercuspation (The Academy of Prosthodontics, 1999). MCP (muscular contact position) is defined by Mohl as follows: The position of the mandible when it has been raised by voluntary muscular effort to initial occlusal contact with head erect. In an asymptomatic individual the muscular contact position will ordinarily be consistent with intercuspal position. One may demonstrate this consistency by noting the ability to accurately and repeatedly tap the teeth directly into the intercuspal position when the head erect (Mohl ND, 1991).

2. INTRODUCTION

When it is required to evaluate whether a patient's habitual occlusion, so called intercuspal position (ICP) is correct or not, a reference position for occlusion is

Kengo Torii

needed. In general dental practice, there is no problem in TMD asymptomatic patients, because the patient's ICP is stable and reproducible. Unless the ICP is stable or reproducible, practitioners cannot treat their patients. However, in the case that the patient's masticatory system is doubtful of pathology in the muscles or TMJ, the practitioner has to determine the correct occlusal position using a reference position. The reference positions are generally classified into the ligamentous position and the muscular position.

3. RETRUDED CONTACT POSITION

Retruded contact position is the ligamentous position and is described as the position which is not influenced by such factors as the position of the head and posture. Krough-Poulsen and Olsson described that the retruded contact position is the most cranial position of the mandible after it has performed a terminal hinge closure. A short, straightforward slide from the retruded contact position (RCP) into ICP seems to be harmonious pattern in most natural human dentitions, both in adults and children. However, interferences which cause the mandible to slide from the RCP into the ICP through an oblique course deviating from a symmetrical movement are commonly considered a cause of functional disturbances of the stomatognathic system (Krough-Poulsen EG & Olsson A, 1966). Ingervall compared RCP in children to adults to elucidate the following questions: (1) Can the retruded contact position of the mandible be determined with the same precision in children as in adults? (2) How large is the difference between retruded contact position and intercuspal position in sagittal, vertical and frontal plane in children with normal occlusion? Do children differ from adults regarding the difference between retruded contact position and intercuspal position? And he summarized as follows: In the functional analysis of malocclusion in association with orthodontic treatment of children the rest position is the position most commonly used as reference. In functional analysis of adults and in prosthetics, however, retruded positions of the mandible are preferred to reference positions. With reference to sagittal positions retruded positions are better than the rest positions. It has, however, been claimed that retruded positions in children may be misleading owing to a greater range of dorsal mobility of the mandible. The group of subject consisted of (a) 36 girls with normal occlusion and with a mean age of 9 years 10 months and (b) 29 dental nurses with mean age of 19 years and 8 months. The retruded contact position of the mandible was recorded with the intra-oral wax record technique. The position of the mandible relative to the maxilla in retruded contact position was determined in the sagittal, vertical and frontal planes by means of roentgencephalometry. Double determinations and sometimes triple determinations were made. The systemic and accidental errors of the method were calculated. The difference between the retruded contact position and intercuspal position was likewise determined in the sagittal, vertical and frontal planes with roentogencephalometric method. The investigation showed that with the method used it is possible to determine the position of the mandible in the retruded contact position with good precision. But in children the most retruded position of the mandible was obtained at second registration. The mean difference in the sagittal and vertical plane between retruded contact position and intercuspal position was the same in the children as in the adults. In the children, however, the mean lateral difference between the two positions was larger than in the adults. The results obtained from the investigation showed that the retruded positions of the mandible in children at 10 years of age can be used as reference positions in functional analysis of occlusion (Ingervall B, 1964). Helkimo *et al.* investigated the variation of RCP and muscular position under different recording conditions, and reported that the errors of recording of the RCP are very minor and do not vary from one examiner to another; the precision of the recording of the muscular position was much lower than that of the RCP. They summarized as follows: The variation of recordings of the retruded position and the muscular position of the mandible was examined with the graphic method (Gothic arch tracing) on 10 men, aged 21 to 26, with complete dentitions. The investigation showed that the errors of recording of the retruded mandibular position are very small and do not vary from one examiner to another. The precision of recording of the retruded position was largely the same whether the recording was made by the terminal hinge movement or by Gothic arch tracing and was not affected by the posture of the subject (sitting or lying) or by the position of the examiner (on right or left side of the subject). The precision was largely the same for determination of the position of the mandible in antero-posterior and medio-lateral direction. The precision of the recording of the muscular position was much lower than that of the retruded position. This was especially the case regarding the position of the mandible in antero-posterior direction. The precision of recording of the muscular position *was not influenced by the posture of the subject* but was lower in antero-posterior than in medio-lateral direction. The position of the mandible in the retruded position did not vary from one examiner to another, but in medio-lateral direction it was influenced somewhat by the position of the examiner relative to the subject (right or left side). The effect in medio-lateral direction was reflected in a shift of the mandible by, on the average, 0.1 mm in direction away from the examiner. The position of the mandible in the retruded position was not appreciably affected by the posture of the subject or by the recording method (by the hinge movement or with the Gothic arch). The position of the mandible in the muscular position varied in antero-posterior direction with the posture of the subject. The most anterior position was noted when the subject was standing and the most posterior when he was lying (mean difference 0.6 mm). Such a difference was also found between the standing and sitting positions (mean difference 0.4 mm). The results show that because of its good reproducibility the retruded position is suitable as a reference position in functional analysis of the occlusion while the muscular position cannot be recommended as a reference position (Helkimo M *et al.*, 1971). In addition, Helkimo and Ingervall investigated the recording methods of the RCP in patients with mandibular dysfunction, and reported that in comparison between passive (applied light pressure to the chin) terminal hinge recordings, active (applied heavy pressure to the chin) terminal hinge recordings and habitual closures, the passive hinge recording showed the best consistency. Moreover, they added the following: Based upon the results of this study, simple instruction on relaxation of the jaw for a passive registration is sufficient to secure a recording of the retruded position of the mandible with clinically acceptable certainly in most situations. The precision of passive recordings of the retruded position with distal pressure has in previous studies of normal patients been found to be considerably higher than for the muscular position and also higher than for recordings with "moderate chin guidance". This finding was also verified in this patient material. The use of the retruded position as a reference position can therefore be recommended also for individuals with mandibular dysfunction symptoms. During the recording the conventional technique with passive hinge movement and a posterior pressure should be used. It is recommended that an occlusal adjustment be checked and readjusted after the symptoms have disappeared. Even if the positional changes before and after treatment of the symptoms were, on the average, small in this material (mean, 0.20 mm), there might in single cases be relatively large differences between the retruded position recorded in an acute stage of symptoms and after treatment. No *extensive* occlusal adjustment or reconstructive work on a patient with acute TMJ muscle-pain dysfunction symptoms until relief of the symptoms has been achieved *e.g.* by the aid of a bite splint. In this study, however, the maximum difference in antero-posterior direction before and after treatment was 0.7 mm and in medio-lateral direction 0.9 mm (Helkimo M & Ingervall B, 1977). Ingervall described that the terminal hinge movement is a border movement and therefore, readily reproducible, and it is a cinematically simple movement and therefore, useful in mounting of casts on the articulator. For mechanical reasons, the articulator can repeatedly guide only purely rotational movements with precision (Ingervall B, 1964). Hobo and Iwata investigated reproducibility of mandibular centricity in three dimensions by bilateral manipulation, Chin-point guidance and unguided closure, and reported that bilateral manipulation showed the most consistent reproducibility and is recommended for centric relation registration (Hobo S & Iwata T, 1985). However, Torii observed various mandibular closures and reported that for the terminal hinge closure in which the mandible was guided by the Chin-point, no statistically constant rotation center was observed; for the most retruded closure of the mandible in which each subject was asked to make the most retruded position by his or her own effort, a constant rotation center was found in two of five subjects; for habitual closure of the mandible no constant rotation center was observed, and where the interocclusal distance was less than 1 mm the mandible seemed to close perpendicular to the occlusal plane (Torii K, 1989). Regarding the occlusal adjustment using retruded contact position as a reference position, Riise (Riise C, 1982) described as follows: The adjustment starts in the supine position with guided closing movements into the retruded contact position (RP), with the patient exerting both light and hard pressure. The recordings in this position are obtained by the common method of guiding the mandible into hinge axis position. According to Ramfjord and Ash (Ramfjord SP and Ash MM, 1966), the best evidence of a correct position is the operator's feeling of a completely relaxed mandible that can easily be moved up and down on the retrusive hinge path into tooth contact. Instructing the patient to use light and hard pressure when the RP contact position is reached, reveals if there are any pivoting effects on the mandible. The adjustment in RP proceeds until no slide is evident. If a slide between RPA (adjusted retruded position) and the intercuspal position is unavoidable, the mandible should move in a purely sagittal direction with bilaterally equal contacts. After RP adjustment is completed, adjustment in free closing movements into intercuspal position follows with the patient, still in the supine position, exerting light and hard pressure until simultaneous, bilaterally equal contacts are established, especially on the posterior and canine teeth. If possible, more favorable directions of forces (axial) are to be established by the adjustment in order to enhance a maintainable occlusal stability. In addition, the stability of the single tooth will be improved. The first adjustment step ends with the patient sitting upright without a headrest and looking straight forward. Then, free closing movements, relaxed and fast, are performed with light and hard pressure and contacts are marked on opposing teeth. Sometimes, minor adjustments slightly anterior to the IPA (intercuspal position) adjusted marking are necessary. The result of the Step I occlusal adjustment will be a series of evenly distributed point contacts in the IPA (intercuspal position adjusted), important not only for occlusal stability but also for constituting the important prerequisite for Step II. For the most part, point contacts will automatically be achieved as a consequence of this method. The Step I occlusal adjustment should be performed only in the upper jaw, regardless if there is a cross-bite. With this restriction to the upper jaw, a little more tooth substance must be sacrificed in some patients. An area in the lower jaw may sometimes be involved. Because the distance between RPA (Retruded position adjusted) and IPA (intercuspal position adjusted) is small in most instances, failure to reduce this area in favor of adjustment in the upper jaw only implies reducing a little more on the upper teeth. This amount is negligible because of the extremely small spots to be adjusted and the small diamonds used. Instead, restriction of adjustment to the upper jaw only implies a simpler, more systemic, and more controllable procedure (Riese C, 1982). Regarding this occlusal adjustment, Tsolka *et al*. reported from their study of double-blind method that a marked placebo effect was demonstrated, together with the difficulties of eliminating slides and non-working interferences in one treatment session, when treatment is provided directly in the mouth (Tsolka P *et al*., 1992). In most normal, natural dentitions, the ICP is located 1 mm forward from the RCP. When the ICP is needed to be newly established somewhere besides the present ICP, how is it able to be established three-dimensionally using the RCP as a reference position for each patient? In addition, as described in Chapter 3, efficiency of occlusal analysis or adjustment using RCP as reference position has not been demonstrated.

4. MUSCULAR CONTACT POSITION

Mohl described that the muscular contact position is the position of the mandible when it has been raised by voluntary muscular effort to initial occlusal contact with the head erect. In an asymptomatic individual, the muscular contact position will ordinarily be consistent with the intercuspal position. One may demonstrate this consistency by noting the ability to accurately and repeatedly tap the teeth directly into the intercuspal position when head is kept straight (Mohl ND, 1991). Brill *et al*. described that the ligamentous position is an *extreme* position; the mandible cannot be displaced more posteriorly than this position, the limiting factor to further retrusion being the lateral ligaments of the joints. This was shown by Posselt (1952) who was not able to retrude the mandible posterior to this position when curare, muscle relaxant, was administered to a patient; he was, however, able to obtain a more backward displacement of the mandible of a cadaver after sectioning the lateral ligament of the joint capsule. The mandible may be retruded to this ligamentous position, either by an active movement of the patient or passively by the operator pressing on the symphysis menti when the patient is relaxed completely. Provided complete relaxation is obtained, this position can be recorded by means of a wax wafer and is reproducible repeatedly because of the permanency of the limiting joint structures. As well as being recordable by a wax wafer this position may be located by the well known Gothic arch tracing. Posselt has shown conclusively that the most retruded jaw position corresponds with the apex of the Gothic arch. From this position, the jaw may be opened, again either actively by the patient after training or passively by the operator, in such a way that there is no protrusive component to the movement. The jaw will be described a "hinge movement", the condyles providing a "hinge axis" for the movement which operates through an average distance of approximately 20 mm measured at the incisor region (Posselt U, 1952). Further opening is accompanied by concomitant forward translation of the condyles in the glenoid fossa. The association of the ligamentous position with hinge opening has led to its being referred to alternatively as the hinge position. However, the author prefers the term ligamentous position because the lateral ligaments of the joints define the position. Only in a few people the ligamentous position does coincide with the tooth position (interdigitated position of teeth). In about 90 per cent of adults the tooth position lies approximately 1mm anterior to the ligamentous position (Posselt U, 1952). During all the different functional movements carried out by the mandible, only during mastication, and then only for a short time when chewing the hardest food, is this ligamentous position utilized. The second position is tooth position. It can be recorded by a wax wafer or by simply interdigitating upper and lower models. However, it is a basic position of the mandible when opposing posterior teeth are present, and naturally, it is absent in the edentulous state. It is a position used recurrently in all categories of jaw movements. Muscular position is controlled by the musculature. In the majority of patients with standing cusped teeth present, the muscular position coincides with tooth position (interdigitated position of teeth). However, in an appreciable number it is not, and in such cases it may be more anteriorly or more posteriorly placed than the tooth position. It is postulated by the authors that the coincidence of the muscular and tooth positions constitutes a physiological condition: where these two positions do not coincide a pathological, or potentially pathological, condition results. In a very few patients all three mandibular positions – ligamentous, tooth, and muscular coincide. In some patients the muscular position of the mandible can always be accurately recorded. However, in others very small antero-posterior variations will occur at the same or on successive sessions. There are some patients, also in whom the muscular position cannot be demonstrated; this does not mean that it does not exist, but a relaxed condition cannot be induced in that particular patient by that operator (Brill N *et al.*, 1959). Regarding the formation of centric relation, Moyers described that the mandible is moved and supported by a group of muscles most of which receive their innervation from the fifth nerve. They are classic examples of antigravity muscles. The postural reflex controlling the position of the mandible against gravity has its synaptic connections in the brain stem in a similar manner to those of the limb and back muscles in the spinal cord. When all the muscles capable of moving the mandible demonstrate no other contractions than those necessary to hold the bone in a balanced position against gravity, a state of equilibrium is maintained. The physiologist calls this the postural position of the mandible. The dentist calls it the physiologic rest position of the mandible. The latter term is a poor one, for the position is no more physiologic than any other mandibular position, and the muscles are not at rest. Postural reflexes are primitive and unlearned. A series of seventeen neonates has been studied during the first three days of postnatal life. It could be demonstrated electromyographically that each child already had a postural reflex. This is not surprising since a starting point is needed for some of the reflex movements of the mandible during sucking, swallowing, coughing, *etc.* Perhaps this is the only postural reflex fully developed so early. Few others would be needed until the infant begins to sit upright, move his limbs, stand and walk. Many of the most highly developed reflexes involving skeletal muscle at birth are concerned with basic matters of survival such as breathing, feeding and protection of the air passage. All such reflexes involve the use of the fifth nerve musculature, with the postural position of the mandible as the starting point for all movements involved. Only the postural position is consistently observed prior to eruption of the teeth. Sillman (Sillman JH, 1948) spoke about the development of an "occlusal sense" as the erupting primary teeth first met their antagonists of the opposite jaw. This "occlusal sense" is the formation of the neuromuscular reflex establishing centric relation. Centric relation has been spoken of as if it was a morphologic trait like big ears or blue eyes. But since it is not present at birth, it must come later, either through learning or the acquirement of neuromuscular features not present at birth. The postural position is easily recorded in the neonate, but repeated efforts to locate centric relation met with failure until the age at which the primary occlusion was established. As the teeth occlude, afferent impulses of touch and pressure are transmitted through the mesencephalic root of the fifth cranial nerve to the brain where they may alter and affect the motor impulses being transmitted to the muscles controlling the position of the mandible. After the teeth have erupted, the muscles learn one position of occlusion providing a maximum of occlusal contact and minimum of torque or lateral stress and strain on the roots of the teeth. This is the beginning of centric relation. The muscles alone could not establish such a mandibular position, while they are contracting. But the intercuspation of the teeth makes it possible for the brain to learn quickly this new mandibular position. Centric relation is established during the early stages of the primary dentition when occlusal anomalies are at a minimum. At the beginning, centric relation and centric occlusion are identical. *Centric relation is the first established neuromuscular reflex concerning mandibular position when the teeth are in occlusion.* The centric relation reflex is controlled not only by the stretch receptors in the muscles of mastication, but by the receptor organ in the periodontal membranes as well. The periodontal receptors demand a high degree of localization of mandibular positioning. It seems important that the postural position is maintained by the myotatic reflex alone, while the centric relation involves both muscles and periodontal membranes for its maintenance. Centric relation involves more neuromuscular activity, since the mandible must be held in elevation above the postural position in a position permitting occlusal harmony. The anteroposterior limits of centric relation are defined first, since the primary incisors erupt first and restrict mandibular movements in this one direction only. Later, the teeth in the lateral segments of the dental arch inhibit mediolateral positioning, and thus help localize the limits of centric relation in this other direction. The least displacement of the mandible, anteroposteriorly or mediolaterally, immediately sets off a shower of afferent impulses which elicit a motoneuron response stabilizing the mandible in these two directions. Greater mandibular displacement is necessary vertically for a similar response to occur. Opening changes in vertical position of the mandible cause only the firing of stretch receptors and do not, of course, cause stimulation of the periodontal receptors. Direct biting pressure in line with the long axes of the teeth has little effect, but the slightest angular vector of force against a tooth elicits a response from the periodontal proprioceptors. This helps explain the more precise limits of centric relation anteroposteriorly and mediolaterally. It also explains why we have somewhat more latitude in changing vertical dimension than in shifting the mandible horizontally. During growth of the craniofacial complex of bones, centric relation must change, for the mandible grows at a faster rate downward and forward than do the maxillae. Centric relation is not the same when one is tensed and tired as when one is freshened and relaxed. It is different when one is afraid than when one is quiet and at ease. Since centric relation is a neurologic concept, the reflexes controlling centric relation must have been learned and be capable of some learning. Both the postural position and centric relation become relatively more stable with age, but the concept of a fixed and immutable centric relation is contrary to all that is known of neuromuscular physiology. Pain in either the dental or the joint region will result in a remarkable and dramatic effect upon the muscle action. The result is usually "splinting" of all the muscles capable of moving the joint. This phenomenon is a continuous contraction of all the muscles in order to immobilize the joint, and thus avoids further pain which might be caused by movement. Perhaps the most intriguing alterations in the basic reflex patterns are those which arise due to altered or impaired occlusal harmony. These changes have great clinical significance from early childhood onwards. As each primary tooth is lost, it is followed by a permanent successor that is different in size and shape from its predecessor. During the mixed dentition stage, occlusal interferences are many, and the muscles must repeatedly learn new pattern of mandibular closure to avoid interfering teeth. The pathways of centric relation, having only been established in the central nervous system for a short time, are not as firmly entrenched as in the adult. The constant adaptation to new stimuli is frustrating to the muscles, hence the difficulties are usually encountered in reliably recording centric relation in children. It is at this time that the muscles frequently adopt an occlusal position that does not coincide with centric relation. It is important to remember that no repeatedly used position of occlusal contact which does not coincide with centric relation is ever acquired by chance. All are learned neuromuscular reflex patterns forced on the masticatory system. These new positions of occlusal contact usually begin as expedient processes for avoiding interferences and providing better function the centric relation offers at the moment. The continued presence of the occlusal disharmony, as in the case of a severe malocclusion, causes the new reflex pattern of pathways to be used so repeatedly that the new position of the mandible may resemble centric relation. This acquired position may be termed "the usual position of occlusal contact". The use of such terms as acquired centric, "new centric", *etc.*, seems ill-advised, for the position is not centric relation. It would also seem redundant to speak of "true centric" or "original centric". The adjective "centric" should be used to refer to one position only. All positions of occlusal contact, other than centric occlusion to which the patient repeatedly returns, are properly and simply termed eccentric occlusal positions. The earlier in life an eccentric occlusion is adopted and used, the firmer the hold on the nervous system, for it is simply a habit. Also, it is more difficult in adulthood to locate centric relation and restore normal masticatory functioning. This is the most forceful argument for eliminating tooth interferences in the primary dentition and for early orthodontic treatment. The effects of these abnormal muscle reflex patterns upon the growth of the craniofacial skeleton are not yet fully known (Moyers RE, 1956). "Centric relation" described by Moyers means muscular contact position, and Torii and Chiwata located this "centric relation" using an anterior flat plane bite plate which disrupts the motor program responsible for guiding the mandible to the habitual occlusal position (the usual position of occlusal contact termed by Moyers) (Torii K & Chiwata I, 2005). Torii and Chiwata called this centric relation; that is muscular contact position, as bite plate-induced occlusal position (BPOP). On the other hand, regarding occlusal adjustment, Watt and MacGregor developed their occlusal adjustment method using the muscular contact position and described the follows: The most retruded position of the mandible is not used in function. The findings of many workers in this field confirm that the intercuspal position is the most important functional position. Investigations with ultra-high-speed cinematography and movement transducers show that during each chewing cycle the mandible pauses 0.24 sec in the intercuspal position. When the intercuspal position does not coincide with the muscle position (*i.e.* the position in which the mandible closes when the muscles are in optimum function), the patient has a malocclusion that is potentially pathological. The clinical problem is to establish a stable intercuspal position that coincides with a physiologically acceptable muscle position. By using the sounds of occlusion to monitor the occlusal correction, you can identify a patient's adaptive response to minor alterations of the occlusion and follow the progress towards occlusal stability. When the occlusion is unstable the teeth hit and slide into the intercuspal position and the sounds are muffled, but when the occlusion is stable the teeth make impact sounds of short duration as they close directly in the intercuspal position without any slide. Once we have established, in the absence of muscle and joint pain, a stable occlusion (Class A) that is recognizable and reproducible by the patient, we have achieved our purpose. To define the position in anatomical terms is virtually impossible, as there may be a number of positions to which the patient can easily adapt and in which a satisfactory stable occlusion can be established. Nevertheless, in our present state of knowledge it would appear that retruded stable positions are generally more satisfactorily than more anterior stable positions, although it is not uncommon to find patients who have used the latter satisfactorily for many years. The clinical necessity of establishing a recognizable position for the mandible appears to oppose consideration of self-regulating nature of physiological function. However, gnathosonic techniques, by enabling us to put occlusion on a time-bas e, can display the adaptive responses of our patients and lead, during the progress of treatment, to the recognition by both dentist and patient of a satisfactory stable intercuspal position. With articulator techniques it is necessary to record at a particular moment, a retruded mandibular position that is then taken as a reference position from which the occlusion is assessed and interceptive contact diagnosed and corrected. However, each small alteration of the teeth is accompanied by an adaptive change in the position of the mandible, which the articulator cannot adequately reflect. As a result the dentist removes much more tooth surface in reducing contacts that intercept closure on the terminal hinge axis than would be necessary if the postural adaptation by the patient was taken into consideration. What has been said so far may appear to be too vague to satisfy proponents of the hinge-axis techniques, but it is nearer to physiological reality. Those who use gnathosonic techniques very soon find that they demand much greater precision than any articulator technique. The gnathosonic record is indeed a hard taskmaster. The method the authors use to detect and remove abnormal contacts in order to establish a stable intercuspal position is as follows: (1) Relieve the patient's symptoms of muscle and joint pain with a temporary occlusal splint on the maxillary arch. This is purely a diagnostic appliance; by removing the cuspal guidance it allows the mandible to occupy the muscle position and hence produces relaxation of the muscles. The splint should present a smooth surface to the mandibular teeth. If possible ensure that the cusp tips of all these teeth contact but do not indent the appliance, so that tooth movement is minimal. Other methods of relaxing the muscles can be used (heat, ethyl chloride spray, injection of local analgesic, biofeedback, physiological pulsing technique). (2) After completing the diagnosis when the muscles are relaxed, start the treatment phase, locating and removing intercuspal contacts. (3) Place the patient in the supine position with the teeth apart, or with the occlusal splint in the mouth, so that no tooth-to-tooth contact takes place (tooth contact would cause the patient to adapt to the malocclusion and this is undesirable at this stage of treatment). (4) Ask the patient to open and close the jaw several times without tooth contact and then, after the splint has been removed, request that the teeth are brought gently together into light contact. Before this, warn the patient to note which tooth contacts first. (5) As the patient closes into contact, listen with the stereostethoscope so that you can confirm on which side the contact occurs. (6) Ask the patient to open the mouth again and place thin articulating paper or occlusal indicating wax on the maxillary teeth. (7) Ask the patient to close gently until the same contact is again felt. Observe this contact and modify the tooth accordingly. (8) Continue with this procedure until you achieve all round stable contact of teeth in this position. Almost invariably the patient notices an improvement when stability is reached. This stability can be checked quite easily with a stereostethoscope. (9) Raise the chair until the patient is in an upright position and correct the occlusion in the same way as previously and stabilize it in this position also. Do not make any attempt to force the jaw into a retruded position, but simply use the posture of the patient to place the mandible in its physiologically retruded position. Only grind one or two contacts at each session as adaptations to the new occlusion take place between sessions. In this way a stable position can be achieved with minimal grinding. This concept of occlusion is closer to the physiological reality than concepts based on the terminal-hinge-axis of the mandible as a reference position. It is helpful to think of the intercuspal position in terms of the 'brain end' of occlusion rather than in terms of the 'dental end'. By this is meant that when a stable reproducible position has been achieved the afferent impulses from periodontium, joints and muscles will produce a reproducible and recognizable engram within the brain which represents the base line from which masticatory activity takes place. We believe that food between the teeth distorts this engram and calls forth the appropriate muscular responses to deal with the food during mastication. However, if a recognizable and reproducible pattern of intercuspal occlusion is not present, the deflective tooth contact also distorts the engram and incoordinated occlusal activity results as shown by large variations in occlusal sound duration. When you have removed abnormal contacts interfering with the path of closure of the mandible into the intercuspal position, repeat the procedure to remove abnormal contacts interfering with the eccentric occlusal positions. It is particularly important to remove premature contacts on the non-working side (overbalancing contacts) as they cause symptoms more often than cuspal interferences on the working side (Watt

DM & MacGregor AR, 1984). Although Watt begins the occlusal adjustment in supine position, the author does not agree with this because the muscular contact position coincides with the intercuspal position when a subject is in an upright position. The occlusal adjustment in the muscular contact position should be started in an upright position. In addition, the author is concerned about that during directly grind premature contact in the mouth, the pass of closure would be deviated from the correct muscular closure on time by time of closing for the adjustment. In the articulator techniques of the author (see Chapter 7), the occlusal analysis is performed on casts mounted on an articulator with muscular contact position record (BPOP record), not with the retruded contact position (hinge axis record) record, and occlusal equilibration would be performed based on the results obtained from the occlusal analysis on the articulator. McNamara described *Median occlusion* using the activity of the masticatory muscles as follows: Occlusal coordination can be examined by asking the patient to open his mandible widely and then snap it shut. In the absence of deflective occlusal contacts this results in an instantaneous, accurate interdigitation into the median occlusal position. This occlusal position is considered the beginning and the end of reflex masticatory movements, and it is here that integrity exists among the dentition, the TMJ, and the controlling neuromusculature. Reflex electromyographic (EMG) silent periods are demonstrated in the masseter and temporal muscles following tooth contact at the physiologic median occlusal position. Furthermore tooth contacts during chewing trigger a pause in the mandibular elevator muscle activity, and after the insertion of balancing-side interferences the number of these EMG silent periods increases. McNamara summarized from the result of his study as follows: An investigation of the neuromuscular effects of dental contact at the physiologic median occlusal position was conducted before and after occlusal adjustments. Eighteen patients with histories of functional disturbances of the masticatory system, but whose painful symptoms had subsided, were analyzed before and after occlusal adjustments. Nine of the patients with missing teeth received fixed partial dentures and occlusal adjustments. Another group of nine subjects with normal occlusions was used as controls. Electromyographic recordings of the bilateral temporal and masseter muscles enabled quantification of two reflex parameters, the EMG silent period duration, and the mechanical latency of the jaw-opening reflex. Phase-plane traces of jaw-closing velocity as a function of position displayed the repeatability of the median occlusal position. The statistical analysis disclosed that mean duration of EMG silent periods and latency of the jaw-opening reflex were significantly reduced following the treatment procedures. Within the limits of this study it was concluded that the described occlusal adjustments will reduce the masticatory reflexes evoked at median occlusal position to within the range of normal subjects. Furthermore these changes can be monitored by electrophysical methods (McNamara DC, 1977). Klineberg also described that median occlusal position (MOP) is a dynamic contact position of the teeth that may be obtained on command by a snap jaw closure following moderate jaw opening. In addition, MOP analysis is carried out as part of clinical occlusal analysis to determine the presence of a clinical discrepancy in jaw support between a retruded jaw position (RP) and the dynamic muscular jaw position (MOP). If such an interocclusal position discrepancy is observed, a slide from RP to ICP and MOP will present, usually with a vertical, lateral and horizontal component. In addition he also described that occlusal analysis of articulated study casts does not show MOP tooth contacts, so that the positional discrepancy on articulated casts will show a slide from RP to IP that will be similar to that existing clinically (Klineberg I, 1991). Jankelson described *Myocentric* induced by transcutaneous electrical stimulation and that inconsistency between the myocentric position and ICP results in mandibular dysfunction (Jankelson B, 1979). However, Cooper *et al.* reported that habitual trajectories and healthy neuromuscular trajectories of movement did not correspond with each other in 19 out of 26 (73%) asymptomatic subjects (Cooper BC *et al.*, 1984). Tripodakis *et al.* compared the reproducibility of three mandibular positions and reported that neuromuscular position (voluntarily closed position) is able to provide adequate reproducibility and can be used as a reference position, they summarized as follows: The investigation was conducted to examine the location and reproducibility of three mandibular positions (CR: centric relation; CO: centric occlusion; NM: neuromuscular position) in relation to body posture (sitting and supine) and the insertion of a mandibular positioning device (before and after). The findings are summarized as follows. 1) CO and NM were located anterior and lateral to CR (mean anterior distance 0.8 mm and mean lateral distance 0.12 mm). 2) The reproducibility of CO was found to be less than that of CR but greater than that of NM. 3) The location and reproducibility of CR were not affected by body posture or the insertion of the mandibular positioning device. 4) The location and reproducibility of CO were not affected by body posture, but were affected by the insertion of the mandibular positioning device, which led to more precise posterior position. 5) The location and reproducibility of NM were slightly affected by posture and greatly affected by the insertion of the mandibular positioning device. In the supine position a more posterior NM was obtained. After the insertion of the mandibular positioning device, NM became as precise as CO and was located anteroposteriorly between CO and CR. Therefore, under the circumstances described in this investigation, NM is able to provide adequate reproducibility and can be used as a reference point in clinical occlusal management. 6) As the experiment proceeded, all records showed an increasing precision in the five levels of replication (Tripodakis A *et al.*, 1995). Calagna *et al.* investigated the influence of four clinically accepted methods of neuromuscular conditioning (Myo-Monitor, Anterior jig, Bilateral occlusal stimulation and Maxillary bite plane) upon the consistency and relative position of centric relation (retruded position) registration, and reported as follows: In all, the bite plane method led to the most retruded results. The mean position for the anterior jig method of conditioning was second most posterior in five cases. The mean position for the Myo-Monitor recordings and bilateral occlusal stimulation recordings gave similar rank orders. In 12 of the 15 subjects, the mean position with free closure (muscular position) was the most anterior. The bite plane method led to the most consistent recordings. In 13 of the 15 subjects, the bite plane method was the most consistent. With the bite plane method, the mean centric relation position averaged 0.70 mm posterior to the centric occlusal position (intercuspal position). In four of 15 subjects, the differences were greater than 1 mm. The difference between mean centric relation position and centric occlusion was about 0.3 mm for the other three methods of conditioning. With free closure, the mean position averaged only 0.1 mm posterior to the centric occlusal position, and was anterior in four of the subjects. With free closure, the mean position averaged only 0.1 mm posterior to the ICP, and anterior in four of the 15 subjects. Based upon results of this investigation, all patients in need of occlusal therapy should receive a minimum of 24 hour bite plane conditioning prior to securing jaw registration (Calagna LJ *et al.*, 1973). Torii and Chiwata observed changes in the habitual occlusal position (HOP) and the bite plate-induced occlusal position (BPOP) in a TMD patient and compared them with changes in severity of symptoms (Torii K& Chiwata I, 2010). *Bite plate-induced occlusal position* (BPOP) is the position obtained during voluntary jaw closing, while in an upright position and after wearing an anterior bite plate for a short time period (Torii K& Chiwata I, 2050). In their case report (Torii K & Chiwata I, 2010), the patient complained pain in the right TMJ area, especially during eating, and a restricted range of jaw motion. An anterior flat plane bite plate was fabricated for him, and the patient was instructed to wear the plate during the day, except when eating or speaking. This appliance therapy was continued until the symptoms were alleviated; meanwhile, the HOP and BPOP were recorded. The statistical significance of the differences between the HOP and BPOP measurements recorded on each day and between two HOP and two BPOP recordings made on different days was calculated using both position factors. The statistical significance of the differences in the variations of the two positions recorded on two different days was also calculated using an ANOVA. In addition, the maximum unassisted opening and pain score on a 10-point Visual Analog Scale (VAS), where 0 denoted "no pain" and 10 denoted "worst pain" were recorded over time. The changes in the symptoms, the discrepancy between the HOP and BPOP value, and the variations in the HOP and BPOP value are shown in Table **1** and Fig. **1**.

Table 1: Changes of the HOP and BPOP, and TMD symptoms on different days

NS	$H_1 B_1$	H_2				H_6	H_7			
S↕										
NS		B_2	$H_3 B_3$	$H_4 B_4$	$H5 B_5$	B_6	B_7	$H_8 B_8$	$H_9 B_9$	$H_{10}B_{10}$
Days	1	3	6	9	12	15	25	33	50	110
VAS	6	3	2	2	0	0	0	0	0	0
Max.	40	42	42	42	42	45	45	45	45	45

NS: Not significant; S: Significant; Days: Days of visits; H_{1-10}: Habitual occlusal position on different days; B_{1-10}: Bite plate-induced position on different days; VAS: Score on a 10-point Visual Analog Scale, where 0 denoted "no pain" and 10 denoted "worst pain"; Max.: Maximum unassisted opening (mm).

On day one, the difference between the HOP and BPOP was not statistically significant. On day 3, however, the difference between the HOP and BPOP at this time-point was significant (p<0.005). The difference between B_1 and B_2 was also significant ($p<0.05$), while that between H_1 and H_2 was not ($p>0.1$). The mean differences between the HOP and BPOP were 0.18 ± 0.14 mm (mediolateral), 0.71 ± 0.68 mm (anteroposterior) and 0.45 ± 0.34 mm (superioinferior). On day 15, the difference between H_6 and B_6 was significant ($p<0.01$), while that between B_5 and B_6 was not significant ($p>0.1$). If this discrepancy had been left untreated, the symptoms would have recurred. Therefore, for ethical reasons, occlusal adjustment was performed for the BPOP after obtaining the patient's informed consent. The discrepancy between H_7 and B_7 was significant, and the patient reported cheek biting on his left side. However, the discrepancy disappeared by day 33, and the cheek biting ceased. The variations in the BPOP values measured on days 25, 33, 50 and 110 were significantly smaller than those measured on day 15 ($p<0.01$) (Fig. **1**). The HOP shifted anterolaterally to the left after occlusal adjustment. The patient's symptoms did not recur during a two-year follow-up period.

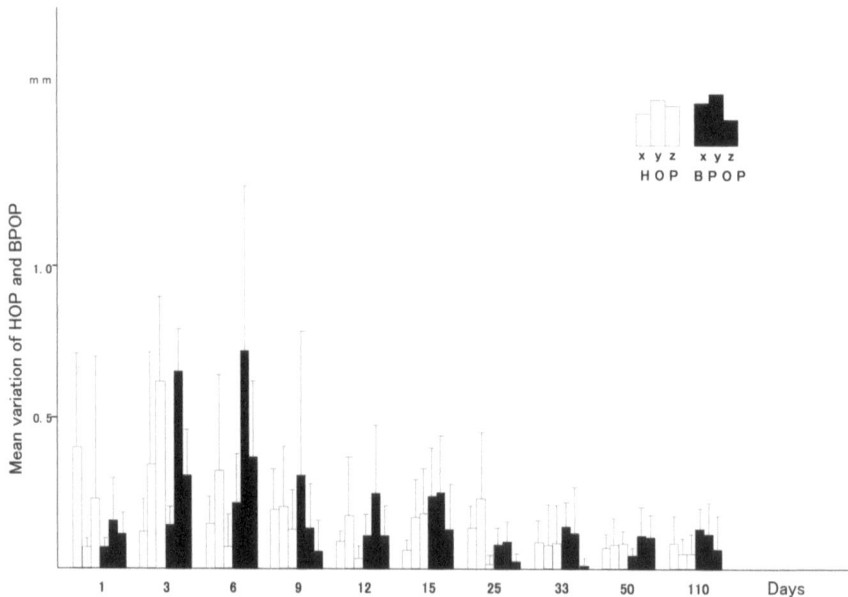

Figure 1: Variations in the HOP and BPOP on different days.

The patient's TMD symptoms completely disappeared after the use of an anterior flat plane bite plate. However, the effect of the plate on the resolution of occlusal discrepancy appeared to be temporary. Therefore, if the patient had not worn the bite plate, the symptoms would have likely recurred. Although the habitually closed position or the muscular contact position has been described as lesser reproducible than the retruded contact position, the variation in the BPOP becomes small after the symptoms disappear.

These results were obtained from a single case. Therefore, these results cannot be applied to every TMD case. However, the variation in the BPOP is expected to decrease according to relieving of symptoms. Provided that the plural BPOP records are confirmed to be consistent by a split cast method, the BPOP is useful as a reliable reference position in occlusal analysis and equilibration.

SUMMARY

The bite plate-induced occlusal position (BPOP) is useful as the reference position of the muscular contact position for occlusal analysis and equilibration. In chapter 5, it will be described how to accurately reproduce the BPOP on an articulator.

REFERENCES

Brill N, Lammie GA, Osborn J, Terry HT (1959). Mandibular positions and Mandibular movements: A review. Brit Dent J 1959;106:391-400.

Calagna LJ, Silverman SI, Garfinkel L (1973). Influence of neuromuscular conditioning on centric relation registrations. *J Prosthet Dent* 1973;30:598-604.

Cooper BC & Rabuzzi DD (1984). Myofascial pain dysfunction syndrome: A clinical study of asymptomatic subjects. *Laryngoscope* 1984;9468-75.

Helkimo M, Ingervall B, Carlsson GE (1971). Variation of retruded and muscular position of mandible under different recording conditions. *Acta Odonotol Scand* 1971;29:423-437.

Helkimo M & Ingervall B (1977). Recording of the retruded position of the mandible in patients with mandibular dysfunction. *Acta Odonotol Scand* 1977;36:167-174.

Hobo S & Iwata T (1985). Reproducibility of mandibular centricity in three dimentions. *J Prosthet Dent* 1985;53:649-654.

Ingervall B (1964). Retruded contact position. *Odont Revy* 1964;15:130-149.

Jankelson B (1979). Neuromuscular aspects of occlusion: effects of occlusal position on the physiology and dysfunction of the mandibular musculature. *Dent Clin North Am* 1979;23:157-168.

Klineberg I (1991). Interarch relationship of teeth, In: *Occlusion: Principles and Assessment,* Klineberg I, pp. (5), Wright, ISBN 072360990X, Oxford.

Krogh-Poulsen WG & Olsson A (1966). Occlusal disharmonies and dysfunction of the stomatognathic system. *Dent Clin North Am* 1966;Nov.:627-635.

McNamara DC (1977). Occlusal adjustment for a physiologically balanced occlusion. *J Prosthet Dent* 1977;38:284-293.

Mohl ND. (1991). Introduction to occlusion, In: *A textbook of occlusion*, Mohl ND, Zarb GA, Carlsson GE, Rugh JD, pp. (15), Quintessence, ISBN0-86715-167-6, Chicago.

Moyers RE (1956). Some physiologic considerations of centric and other jaw relations. *J Prosthet Dent* 1956;6:183-194.

Posselt U (1952). Studies in the mobility of the human mandible. *Acta Odontol Scand* 1952;(Suppl. 10):20-150.

Ramfjord SP & Ash MM (1966). Locating and marking the initial tooth contact in centric relation, In: *Occlusion,* Ramfjord & Ash, pp. (191), Saunders, Philadelphia.

Riise C (1982). Rational performance of occlusal adjustment. *J Prosthet Dent* 1982;48:319-327.

Sillman JH (1948). Serial study of occlusion (Birth to 10 years of age). Am J Orthodontics 1948;34:969-979.

The Academy of Prosthodontics (1999). *Glossary of Prosthodontic Terms.* 7-th ed. St. Louis: C.V. Mosby Co., 1999.

Torii K (1989). Analysis of rotation centers of various mandibular closures. *J Prosthet Dent* 1989;61:285-291.

Torii K & Chiwata I (2005). Relationship between habitual occlusal position and flat bite plane induced occlusal position in volunteers with and without temporomandibular joint sounds. *J Craniomandib Pract* 2005;23:16-21.

Torii K & Chiwata I (2010). A case report of the symptom-relieving action of an anterior flat plane bite plate for temporomandibular disorder. *The Open Dentistry Journal*, 2010;4:218-222.

ISSN:1874-2106.

Tripodakis AP, Smulow JB, Mehta NR, Clark RE (1995). Clinical study of location and reproducibility of three mandibular positions in relation to body posture and muscle function. *J Prosthet Dent* 1995;73:190-198.

Tsolka P, Morris RW, Preiskel HW (1992). Occlusal adjustment therapy for craniomandibular disorders: A clinical assessment by a double-blind method. *J Prosthet Dent* 1992;68:957-964.

Watt DM & MacGregor AR (1984). Preparation of the mouth for removable partial dentures, In: *Designing partial dentures,* Watt DM, MacGregor A R, pp. (205), Wright, ISBN:0 7236 0810 5, Bristol.

CHAPTER 5

Reproducibility of the Muscular Contact Position

Abstract: The reproduction of a habitual (natural) closing movement is considered to be important because this closing movement ends at the muscular contact position (MCP), otherwise known as the intercuspal position (ICP). This closing movement was originally regarded as a hinge-like movement. However, since it has been demonstrated to be a bodily movement, that is, a vertical movement, this vertical movement can be reproduced on an articulator.

Keywords: Hinge-like movement, bodily movement, border movement, habitual movement, rest position, terminal hinge position, intercuspal position, muscular contact position, incisal point, face-bow, check-bite, hinge axis locating, condyle, rotation center, occlusal plane, articulator.

1. TERMINOLOGY

The intercuspal position (ICP) is the maximal ICP. This represents the complete intercuspation of the opposing and is sometimes referred to as the best fit of the teeth, both regardless of the condylar position. It is also referred to as maximal intercuspation (The Academy of Prosthodontics, 1999). The muscular contact position (MCP) is defined by Mohl as follows: "The position of the mandible when it has been raised by voluntary muscular effort to initial occlusal contact with the head erect". In an asymptomatic individual, the MCP will ordinarily be consistent with the ICP. This consistency can be demonstrated by noticing the ability to accurately and repeatedly tap the teeth directly into the ICP when the head is erect (Mohl ND, 1991).

2. INTRODUCTION

Many studies have been performed to investigate various mandibular movements so as to accurately reproduce the intraoral occlusal relationship on an articulator. Initial studies were focused on opening and closing movements of the mandible in the sagittal plane. The mandible can open and close in both protruded and retruded positions. Posselt studied the mobility of the human mandible and summarized the results. Posselt's investigation was comprised of 3 main sections:

(1) the capacity of the mandible for movement, (2) the influence of various factors on the retruded and habitual positions of the mandible, and (3) the relations in the sagittal plane between the retruded (direct or indirect) contact positions, the rest position, and the ICP. The study population was comprised of 65 male dental students aged 20-29 years. All subjects had complete or almost complete dentition. In addition, registrations were made us of a fresh (nonpreserved), edentulous, post-mortem preparation of an elderly male. Graphical model registration and /or profile radiography were used to examine movement in the subjects. Movement paths and positions were analyzed chiefly in the median plane, or in a projection in the sagittal plane. (1) Examination of the mandible's capacity for movement comprised registrations of both active and passive extreme movement paths of the mandible in three subjects. The movement areas obtained in the case of active movements were then compared to those found after passive movements. In addition, the comparison included movement areas obtained by means of registration in a subject under anesthesia and after injection of curare, as well as in a post-mortem preparation. The movement area in the sagittal plane was examined in 15 subjects by means of graphical registration combined with profile radiography. (2) The influence of various factors on the retruded and habitual positions of the mandible was determined in 29 subjects with a posterior bite-opening of 2.6 ± 0.8 mm. In another group comprising 15 subjects, two retruded positions were compared at a degree of bite-opening of 11.8 ± 1.8 mm. (3) Analysis in the sagittal plane of four mandibular positions was performed by means of two points on the mandible: an indicator point at the infradentale and a second point called the articulare, in which the radiograph in the ICP was marked conjointly for both necks of the mandible. Positional changes of the articulare in each individual case were transferred to the film showing the other mandibular positions. Posselt reported the results as follows. (1) The shape of the movement area in the sagittal seems to be characteristic of an individual subject and varies among individuals. The same applies to the movement area in the horizontal plane, provided the movements are recorded with the same degree of posterior bite opening. The border movement parts seem to be reproducible in an individual subject. (2) It was shown that the mandible can perform a posterior hinge-opening and hinge–closing movement. (3a) In the course of the posterior hinge-opening movement, the condyle could be passively prevented from sliding forwards, at

least with a posterior bite opening of 19.2 ± 1.9 mm. If the opening exceeded 25.8 ± 2.2 mm, a forward-downward shift of the condyle occurred, which was also observed if the mandible was passively retruded as much as possible. After some exercise, the subjects were able to actively perform a posterior hinge-opening movement. (3b) The habitual path of closure seems to follow a course anterior to the posterior path. This was observed in all sections of the investigation. The influence of various factors on the retruded and habitual positions of the mandible was as follows. (3c) When the mandible is at the arrow point, the relationship to the point of recording pin is an average 0.1 mm anterior to the position of the same point in the course of a passive hinge-closing movement with a posterior bite-opening of 2.6 ± 0.8 mm. No difference could be demonstrated in the case of a posterior bite-opening of 11.8 ± 1.8 mm. This indicates that, practically, the arrow point relation can be considered equal to the intermaxillary relation during the posterior hinge-movement. (4) The point of the recording pin was not displaced farther posteriorly than the arrow point in any of the cases examined. It could not be shown that a retruded position of the mandible was influenced by traction of chin straps. (5) It could be shown that the arrow point relation of the point recorded was influenced to a negligible degree (averaging 0.05 mm) by the inclination of the head in the sagittal plane. (6) The positions obtained by means of habitual closing movements are moved farther posteriorly when the head and/or the trunk are reclined, although they do not then become maximally retruded positions. The results described in (3b) to (6) above have been established statistically. (7) The relations in the sagittal plane of the retruded (direct or indirect) contact positions, the rest position, and the ICP vary between individuals. The anteroposterior distance between the retruded and ICPs averages 1.25 ± 1.0 mm. In 12 % of the 50 cases examined, the ICP and the maximally retruded direct contact position coincided at the indicator point at the infradentale, the *id*. The point termed the articulare, the *a* (*ip*), coincided with the two positions in 40 % of the cases. The rest position does not seem to be a posterior border position, and the ICP is more rarely so. A shift of the mandible from the rest position to the ICP generally involves a bodily movement of the mandible. (8) With different degrees of posterior bite opening in general it has, been possible to demonstrate differences between border movements and positions and habitual movements and positions. *It has been found that, in principle, the mandible's border movements differ among individuals in their range and directions but are reproducible in a single individual. The habitual movements, however, also seem to vary among individuals* (Posselt U, 1952). Among the various opening and closing movements, so-called natural (habitual) opening and closing movements were focused as functional movements. This was so because the end of closing path should coincide with the ICP and the functional closing path ends at the terminal position that is the ICP. Glickman *et al.* performed a study to determine where the jaw functioned and how the teeth interrelated using a telemetry system. They arrived at the following conclusions: (1) the patient chewed and swallowed with teeth in her existing centric occlusion position (ICP), (2) the prostheses made to coincide with the patient's pre-existing centric occlusion position (ICP) did not alter this pattern of tooth contacts in tests after 36 hours and three weeks wear, (3) the prosthesis with intercuspation in centric relation (terminal hinge position) did not significantly alter the tendency for tooth contacts to occur in the patient's previously existing ICP, (4) the patient had a great difficulty in achieving maximum intercuspation when allowed to close freely with the prosthesis designed to intercuspate in centric relation (terminal hinge position), (5) the use of the terminal hinge in oral rehabilitation is subjected to question because it appears that the patient will not function in this position. Its use as a reference position is doubtful because the distance to the existing centric occlusion position (ICP) is variable and unpredictable (Glickman I *et al.*, 1974). On the other hand, Brill *et al.* stated that the most important vertical position of the mandible is the *rest position* and this position is considered to have a consistency which makes it a reproducible position of reference. In addition, it is appropriate to comment on the nature of the movement from the *rest position* to the tooth position (MCP) (Brill N *et al.*, 1959). The bite plate-induced occlusal position (BPOP) is the MCP and is obtained as the end of habitual closure.

3. HABITUAL OPENING AND CLOSING MOVEMENTS OF THE MANDIBLE

Many studies were undertaken to identify the center of rotation of habitual opening and closing movements. From observations of tracings of the opening and closing movements at the incisal point in humans, and according to the structure of the human temporomandibular joint (TMJ), these movements were shown to be a hinge movement with the center of rotation in the condyle. In fact, many articulators have the mechanism of hinge movement centered around the condyle, and this concept has changed little from its early history until modern times (Mitchell DL & Wilkie ND, 1978). Consequently, ever since the Snow face-bow was developed (McCollum BB, 1939), the positional relationship between the condyle and the dentition, which was regarded as the center of rotation of the opening and closing movements, was transferred by the face-bow to the positional relationship of the rotation axis (condylar shaft) of an articulator and that of the dentition model. Even if it is necessary to change the vertical dimension on an articulator, it should be possible to obtain an occlusal contact relation between the upper and lower teeth of an accurate ICP on an articulator. Therefore, the face-bow is widely used. However, McCollum used an arbitrary condyle point to position models on an articulator with a face-bow, obtained a check-bite (interocclusal record) with the mouth open and mounted the mandibular cast, increased the vertical dimension on the articulator, and allowed the casts to occlude. He observed that when prosthesis was fabricated, inserted into the mouth, and allowed to occlude, there was either a premature contact in the posterior molar area or separation. This may have been caused by the mislocating of the center of rotation of the opening and closing movements (McCollum BB, 1939). Subsequently, the hinge axis locating method was developed, which became a popular method for accurately finding the center of rotation. However, when this method was initially developed, the opening and closing movements performed by a patient to find the center of rotation were apparently habitual opening and closing movements, and because McCollum's article regarding opening and closing movements was vague, did not show any scientific data, and included no reference literature, these movements were misunderstood as opening and closing movements in the most retruded position, and leading to significant confusion (McCollum BB, 1960). Regarding determination of the hinge-axis, McCollum described this as follows: The clutch is adjusted to the teeth, the facebow bar is attached to the projecting stud with a toggle joint, and the arms placed so that they carry the caliper pins in the neighborhood of tragi, one on either side. The patient is told to "let the mouth drop open". Then a rhythmic closing and "dropping open" is established and behavior of the caliper pin is noted. If the point is off the axis, a characteristic arc of movement will be formed by the point of the pin. The actual axis is, of course, at the crossing of the radii of that arc, which, after a little experience, may be estimated almost accurately by the operator. The pin is then moved to this apparent center and the rhythmic "dropping open" and closing of the mouth is repeated. Any error will be noted and new adjustments will be made until there is no arcing of the point but only practically invisible rotation (McCollum BB, 1939). In addition, regarding centric relation, McCollum described the movement as follows. The movements of the mandible are in three dimensions: (1) up and down, (2) forward and back, and (3) right and left. All these movements have a common starting point, which is known as the centric relation. There is even some controversy about this starting point. I define it as "the most retruded positions of the *idle* condyle in the glenoid fossa". Even the anatomic form of the joint indicates that this concept is correct. I do not believe that it is possible to retrude the mandible beyond the normal centric position, except by extreme pressure or a blow by which the joint is injured. Any boxer can testify that the resistance of the joint is sufficient to pass the effect of the blow on to the brain. I do know, however, that whenever the articulation or occlusion of the teeth did not conform to my definition of the centric relation (the most retruded position of the *idle* mandible), there was the characteristic untoward result (McCollum BB, 1960). These movements were misunderstood as opening and closing movements in the most retruded position (as mentioned by Posselt in 1952), and subsequently confusion was the order of the day. On the other hand, studies to find the center of rotation in habitual opening and closing movements have been conducted for a long time. Luce described the method used as follows: A bright silver bead was fastened to a wooden pin or dowel, which was firmly inserted between the inferior central incisors with the subject in a strong sunlight so that a bright spot should be reflected from the bead, a pure profile or side view was photographed, and the sensitive plate was exposed during the opening of the mouth. The bright spot reflected from the bead during the motion was continuously photographed and its excursion recorded on the negative as a line, giving the actual movement of the place upon the jaw to which the bead was opposed. By referring to the records, it will be noticed that the condyle begins to move forward immediately, and even in a small opening of the mouth, it achieves a considerable excursion, contrary to the assertion of Gray and others that with small opening, the condyles simply rotate on a transverse axis against the fibrocartilages (Luce CE, 1889). Ulrich used the similar method to that employed by Luce and reported as follows. *Instantaneous Axes of the Opening movement,* the marked positions were connected with a straight line for each subject. Then, the position of the kinematic axis for each successive shift of position was mathematically calculated. This method was used as a check on the instantaneous axes constructed geometrically. The main conclusion obtained from these calculations and constructions was that because the condyles start their forward movement immediately upon jaw opening, only a changing axis can be responsible for the opening movement. No single axis could be shown. The paths of an opening and closing movement in the same individual did not coincide. The closing path was generally in front of the opening path when the teeth were not brought together. *Possibility of a Terminal Hinge Opening,* three of the subjects were asked to hold the mandible back in maximal mouth opening. Two of the individuals could not suppress the forward movements of the condyles, but the third individual did achieve an opening movement to almost half of its extent without any significant forward glide of the condyles (Ulrich J, 1959). Bennett aimed to identify a fixed center of rotation in the mandibular movements and described the results as follows: our experiments were conducted especially with reference to the supposedly fixed center of rotation; there is no such point. If experiments similar to those that I have described were made on another individual, the paths of the condyle and symphysis would doubtlessly be found in somewhat different form, and the centrodes necessary to reproduce the movement would also be different; but a single center of rotation for any individual could be quite impossible, unless his condyle never left its position of occlusion, and then it would be in the condyle itself; or unless the paths of the condyle and symphysis were arcs of concentric circle, and this would involve very abnormal anatomical configuration. I will now indulge in a few speculations as to the bearing of what I have said on the possibility of constructing an ideal articulator. In the first place, it would be necessary to obtain several correlative positions of both condyles and some other point in a simpler way than the one adapted, even though less accurate. It is conceivable that this might be done by means of a number of bites of different heights, each with an outside framework to register the several positions of the condyles. From these, the centrodes from which to reproduce the movements can be reproduced and a working articulator may possibly be constructed to imitate nature. Secondly the models of the jaws must be attached to the articulator in such a way that they bear the same positions relative to the line passing through the two condyles as the jaws themselves. This may be done with the face-bow in connection with any one of the bites taken. In this way, it may be possible to reproduce the natural movement of any individual mandible, but there would yet remain the question of finding the correct height of the bite and the correct plane of occlusion. These two considerations are really distinct from the question of the construction of an ideal articulator and are connected with the fact that in edentulous and many other cases, the disease has destroyed the normal conditions. After all, I do not feel at all conceived that the ideal natural articulator is a *sine qua non* for practical prosthetic dentistry. In constructing artificial dentures, we are concerned only with the smallest degrees of opening and with lateral movements with the teeth in occlusion, and I believe that for these purposes, a small movement of rotation and translation combined with some lateral freedom of the correct kind would probably be sufficient if there was a scientific method of fixing the plane of occlusion in relation to the condyles when the normal occlusion has been lost. On this point, I hope to have something to say at a later time, but, as several years have elapsed since I made the experiments which I have only now described, I am able to assure you that you need to have no fear of being in troubled before a somewhat remote date (Bennett NG, 1958). It was evident that these movements were not pure hinge movements around the center of rotation of the condyle, but was complex movements in which the center of rotation shifted with changes in the amount of opening, as it was noted by Charles (Charles SW, 1925; Clapp GW, 1952; Posselt U, 1952; Shanahan TE & Leff A, 1962). Charles summarized his findings as follows: In the normal resting position, the teeth are separated, the mandible having dropped slightly; it has not rotated upon a transverse axis passing through the condyles. The mandible is not depressed by the action of the so-called depressors (genio-hyoid, digastric and platysma). It is depressed and elevated by the interaction of the four muscles, namely the external pterygoid, masseter, internal pterygoid, and temporal, which act as a group. These muscles are arranged in such a way that they hold the mandible in a sling, and, when in action, are so arranged that the action of one portion (depression or elevation) is always opposed by the opposite portion of the group. The result is a controlled, balanced, and rhythmic movement. The condyle does not act as a fulcrum or hinge about which the movements of the mandible take place, and at no time is the condyle in the most posterior part of the fossa. As the action of the depressor group is to draw the head of the condyle forward, it follows that on the slightest separation of the teeth, the condyle has travelled forward and downward from its position of rest (Charles SW, 1925). Clapp summarized the situation, quoting from Gysi's study as follows: The rotation axes in the straight opening movement are far below and behind the entire mandible. The only rotation axis that falls within the border of the mandible is that for the 4-5 segment, the path of extreme opening. The inframandibular muscles activate the straight opening movement. The external pterygoid muscles do not. All the axes for this movement, except the one for extreme opening, are located outside the mandible (Clapp GW, 1952). Posselt summarized as follows: It was shown only in a small number of cases that the ICP is a border position. In other words, in the majority of cases, it seems as if the mandible can be retruded from its ICP. This is in accordance with the results arrived at by Hildebrand (1931), Björk (1947), and Heath (1949) on the basis of clinical measurements made in the incisal part of the mandible. It is,however, difficult by means of direct measurements in a subject to show that a point on the mandible, *e.g.*, the infradentale, moves caudally and posteriorly at the same time and that minor changes in position of points on the condyles are also difficult to demonstrate clinically. The view of the McCollum School that the intercuspal position normally is, and at any rate should be, identical with the arrow point contact position and should thus represent a border position is not confirmed by the results found in my series. That the ICP is no border position and does not seem to force the mandible into border paths corresponds to the mode of function of most of the other joints in the organism, which are generally considered to work through non-extreme positions and not in border paths. In the course of my investigations, I did not intend to deal with the views put forward by Thompson et Brodie (1942) and Thompson (1943, 1946, 1949)) about the rest position and the rest facial height. But my first and foremost aim was to elucidate whether the rest position is a border position or not and to demonstrate its relation in the sagittal plane to the other positions that were recorded. In order to get some idea of the size of the interocclusal (freeway) space measured according to the same method as was used by the authors mentioned above, I made duplicate exposures in 25 subjects of my series and repeated these observations after the course of 6 to 11 months. The average size of the interocclusal (freeway) space proved to be 2.5 ± 1.5 mm. The error of the method was calculated to be 0.6 mm and the actual individual variation was 0.6 mm. The size of the interocclusal (freeway) space shows good conformity with the average vertical (*i.e.*, at right angles to the *n-s* line) distance between the positions of the *id* in the ICP and the rest position as calculated in 50 individuals. This distance was computed to be 2.5 ± 1.25 mm.

Regarding the path of movement between the rest position and the ICP, Thompson (1946, 1949) considered that the closing movement from the rest position to the ICP should normally take place as a rotation around a transverse axis through the condyles, causing the gnathion to move upward and forward. He characterizes an "abnormal path of closure", whereby that the condyles are caused to make sliding movements because of cusp interference, most often posteriorly and cranially. The other examinations which have been made, broadly speaking, shown that in Class I (Angle) occlusion, the condyles perform a rotatory movement or a "primarily rotary movement" in connection with a slight "sliding movement". In cases of Class II (Angle) occlusion, the condyles perform sliding movements of different degrees. I do not consider it possible to compare the abovementioned results with mine, *inter alia* because the investigations referred to involved children, children and adults, or individuals whose age group was not mentioned. Futhermore, I did not undertake any classification of my series into different types of bite and the like for the purpose of examining whether the results may be dependent on them. My investigations have shown that the greatest change of position both of the *id* and of the *a* (*x*) from the intercuspal position to the rest position takes place in a caudal direction and that the average degree of displacement of the two points (irrespective of the direction) is 2.5 mm and 1.4 mm respectively. I can only consider that these results show that the mandible performs a bodily movement between the two positions. The axis of such a movement cannot, at any rate, pass through the condyles. The type of movement that, according to the statements above, has been termed as the normal one, therefore, as a rule, has not been found in my series. My results show a better conformity with those of Chissin (1906) and Bennett (1908) who consider that sliding movements of the condyles occur immediately at the beginning of the habitual opening movement, and also with Higley et Logan's (1941) finding that 70.6 % young adults performed a sliding movement ("forward shift") of the condyles from the ICP to "approximately physiologic rest" (2 mm's opening). Donovan (1950) found a "vertical drop" of the condyles in 20 out of 25 children; nevertheless, they considered that a "rotary movement" was normal in adults. In most cases, the recorded change of position of the *id* from the rest position to the ICP seems to be directed much more upwards and vertically in relation to the *n-s* linet compared with the path of the posterior hinge-movement. The "path" of the *id* from the rest position to the ICP does not, in any case, coincide with the posterior path of closure. The "normal" path of closure from the rest position is considered to be a hinge-movement with its axis through both condyles in many cases, and it has been identified with the posterior hinge-movement. The abovementioned results of my investigations show the different course and character of these two paths of movement. The direction of the change of position of the *id* from the rest position to the ICP shows considerable individual variations, and it was directed upwards and backwards in relation to a line vertical to the *n-s* line in 14 patients (28%). Boman (1948) found a similar direction of the movement path in 12 % of 25 "individuals possessing normal or nearly normal occlusion of the teeth". I have, however, not attempted to elucidate whether such a direction should be due to cusp interference which should force the condyles back into the mandibular fossa when the mandible slid into its ICP. I would only point out that even in the relatively great number of patients whom I have recorded a considerable cranial displacement of the *a* (*x*), this point is generally displaced farther in cranial and posterior directions when the mandible is brought into the retruded direct contact position (Posselt U, 1952). Shanahan and Leff obtained photographic recordings in the normal opening and closing movements of the mandible from both the side and front and reported following findings: The lines appeared to be in the form of arcs in the side view tracings. However, none of these pseudo arcs had a radius that terminated in the region of the condyle. The muscles exercise marvelous control over the mandible during opening and closing movements and mastication. None of the vertical movements lend credence to the existence of a natural mandibular axis. The term artificial mandibular axis designates an axis that is the result of forcing the mandible backward. This axis cannot be found during normal physiologic mandibular movements. An artificial mandibular axis can be produced in one of two ways: the patient may voluntarily retrude the mandible as far as possible during the opening and closing movements or the dentist can apply firm, backward pressure to the chin during the movements. The unusual strain involved in forcing the mandible backward is apparent in the photographs of the movements of the lights during voluntary retrusion. The muscles of the face and neck are taut. The tracing from the side appears irregular. The tracing from the front also gives a clear indication of the patient's struggle to move the mandible back to its most retruded position. However, there was a definite indication that the mandible did open and close on an axis located in the region of the condyles during the retrusive movements. A study of the tracing of the natural opening, closing, and masticating movements of the mandible does not show the presence of a mandibular axis in the region of the condyle (Shanahan EJ & Leff A, 1962). Thompson observed habitual closing movements from the so-called resting position of the mandible to the ICP on cephalometric radiographs and summarized the following findings. 1) The position here referred to a resting position determined by a balance of the musculature that suspends the mandible. It is not affected by either the presence or absence of teeth. This position alone determines the height of the face. 2) The difference between the height of the face when the mandible is at rest and that when the teeth are in occlusion is determined by the amount of space between the upper and lower teeth when the mandible is at rest. This, which is called the free-way space, measures 2-3 mm on an average in a normal dentition. In an abnormal dentition, it may measure 10 mm. or more. 3) The normal closing path of the mandible from the resting to the occlusal position was a hinge movement centered on the lower half of the TMJ because the condyle did not translate. 4) In some individuals, the path of closure is found to be abnormal because of occlusal interference. In these cases, the mandible may be displaced during deglutition and mastication (Thompson JR, 1946). Using similar investigation method, Alexander reported the following. 1) The movement of the condyle when the mandible moves from the rest position to initial contact and full occlusion through an acceptable freeway space with the patient sitting in an upright position may be rotatory or translatory. 2) From the point of initial contact to full occlusion, where there was no cuspal interference, no movement of the condyle was exhibited. 3) In the cases studied showing no displacement, the type of movement shown was the same for both condyles of the same patient. 4) The 5 cases showing a movement of the condyle from initial contact to full occlusion were indicative of cuspal interference. 5) The cases indicative of a displacement did not show the corresponding movement for both the right and left condyles of the same patient when the mandible moved from the rest position to initial contact and then to full occlusion. 6) Roentgenographically, evidence for the proximity of the anterosuperior surface of the condyle to any surface of the eminence was not sufficient to draw any conclusions (Alexander PC, 1952). In contrast, Nevakari performed a study using cephalometric radiography to ascertain whether the movement of the mandible from the rest position to the occlusal position is a pure hinge movement with the axis through the condyles, and if not, whether it deviates from a pure hinge movement. He summarized the following finding. 1) In the cases examined herein, the movement of the mandible from the rest position to the occlusal position has never been a pure hinge movement with the axis through the condyles. 2) The geometrically constructed theoretical axis for the said movement has, in all subjects, been situated outside the condyle, and its location has exhibited considerable individual variation. On the average, the axis of the movement has been located near the processus mastoideus. 3) Upon the mandible's closing from the rest position, the deviation from a pure hinge movement measured at the canine point has on the average been about 1 mm in the distal direction. 4) The condyle has, in all subjects, also undergone a translatory movement, the magnitude of this movement upon the mandible's closing from the rest position being an average of 1 mm backward and upward. 5) The direction of the path of closure measured at the canine point is an average of 11° in relation to a perpendicular of the Frankfort plane, or upward and slightly forward (Nevakari K, 1956). Higley and Logan also investigated the movement of the condyle in mouth opening using radiography and reported the following findings. 1) In all studied subjects, as the mandible dropped from physical rest to an opening of 15 mm, there was a retrusive movement of the chin point. 2) In all subjects, the head of the condyle dropped progressively from physical rest to opening of 15 mm. 3) The majority of subjects (70.6 %) showed a forward shift of the head of the condyle from physical rest to approximately physiological rest. With an opening of 10 mm, 95 % subjects showed a forward shift of the head of the condyle. When the mandible was opened 15 mm, all the subjects showed a forward shift of the head of the condyle. Except one, all subjects showing a distal movement of the head of the condyle presented some tooth interference, which may have caused the assuming of a convenience bite (forward position of the mandible, and, consequently, condyles) in the physical rest position. This may explain the distal shift of the head of the condyles in the first phases of opening. 4) Although the incisal opening never exceeded 12 mm. (approximately half an inch), with this opening 100 % subjects showed both a vertical and a horizontal shift of the head of the condyle. Moreover, in many subjects, the condyle head had moved to a position below the eminentia articularis (Higley LB & Logan RA, 1941). Brown discussed the problem of movements that no conventional articulator reproduces or imitates as follows: The menisci, also called the interarticular fibrocartilages and the interarticular disks, are concavoconvex disks of a cartilaginous nature, functioning between the condyles and the glenoid fossa. Their centers are deeply depressed, forming sockets in which the condyles rest. Their inner and anterior edges are thick compared with their outer and posterior edges. They are resilient and compressible; therefore, two movements of the mandible are allowed, for which, I think, no articulator reproduces or imitates. The first of these movements might be called as the superretrusive movement. It is the movement of the condyles backward and downward from their normal centric positions. When the mandible is in centric relation, the condyles are in their most retruded rest, or unstrained, positions in the fossa, but by greater effort, or straining, the condyles can be forced to positions slightly backward and downward, describing the superretrusive movement. As stated, the movement is made possible by the compressibility of the tissues of the glenoid fossa. It is a strained position, not a normal functional position; therefore, it is not the one in which we as denture prosthesists are greatly interested. The second movement made possible by the resiliency or compressibility of the interarticular tissues is of considerable importance to us. It is known as the intrusive movement, a movement of the condyle of either side upward from its rest position, and it results from the contraction of the powerful temporal and masseter muscles, which drive the condyles bodily into the slightly yielding menisci. It is frequently associated with a slight forward or backward component. The range of movement is short, probably never exceeding one thirty-second inch, though quite sufficient to change the position of applied force on dentures. While it would be a comparatively easy matter to incorporate this movement in an adaptable articulator, I do not know that it has ever been done; nor would it seem to be necessary. It would necessitate making two sets of checkbites, one set under zero pressure and the other under biting stress. I believe that this movement can be accounted in a simpler and an equally effective manner, by making provision for it and by conducting the entire process of denture construction under functional conditions. This means that impressions and checkbites must be made under closed-mouth conditions, and, as nearly as possible, under unvarying pressure throughout. Incidentally, following this technique nullifies, to a large extent, the anterior component of force. If impressions and checkbites are made under working conditions, we need to have a little concern about any slight variation of articulation taking place under zero pressure. Functional efficiency is our goal, and it can be reached through a careful technique, perhaps, with even more certainty than would be possible with an articulator made to reproduce the intrusive movement, since, in the latter case as stated, we would have to contend with inaccuracies inherent in two sets of checkbites (Brown AH, 1930). Torii observed three mandibular closures (terminal hinge closure, most retruded closure and habitual closure). In his study, wax interocclusal records obtained from five subjects during three types of mandibular closing movement at various degrees of jaw opening were successively placed between upper and lower casts that were mounted on an articulator. Recording pins inserted into the lateral sides of the casts were used to record the amount of movements (Figs. **1** and **2**). The rotation centers were calculated and the following results were obtained.

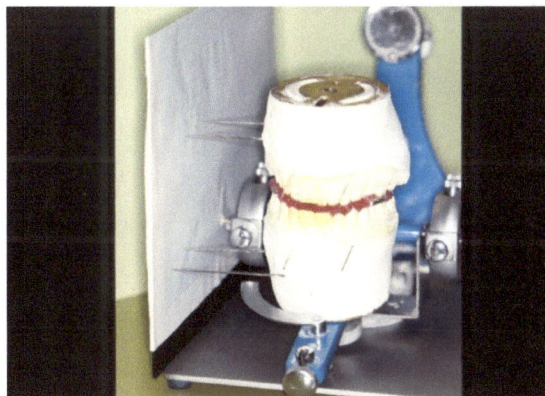

Figure 1: Sagittal plane recording pin position.

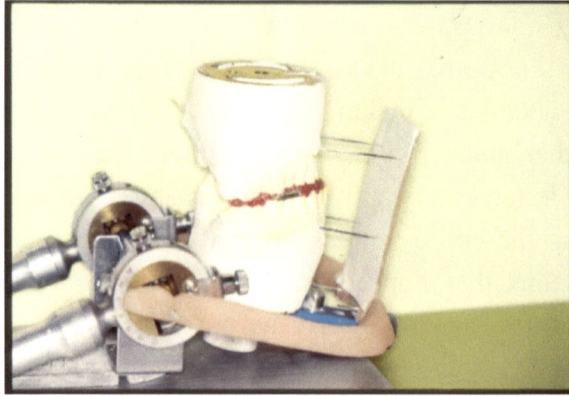

Figure 2: Frontal plane recording pin position.

(1) For the terminal hinge closure (THC) in which the mandible was guided by chin-point, no statistically constant rotation center was observed (Fig. **3**).

(2) For the most retruded closure (MRC) of the mandible in which each subject was asked to adopt the most retruded position by his or her effort, a constant rotation center was found in two of the five subjects (Fig. **4**).

(3) For habitual closure (HC) of the mandible no constant rotation center was observed, and where the interocclusal distance was less than 1 mm, the mandible seemed to close perpendicular to the occlusal plane (Figs. **5** and **6**) (Torii K, 1989).

The HC result indicates that, when the interocclusal distance between the maxilla and the mandible is less than 1 mm in habitual closure, the mandible becomes parallel to the occlusal plane. This 1-mm distance is the usual thickness of a wax bite, and because the thickness of the wax bite cannot be zero according to Millstein *et al*. (Millstein PL *et al*., 1971), a space that corresponds to the thickness of the wax bite in the occlusal plane will always remain after removing the wax record while mounting the upper and lower casts on an articulator with wax bite. That this space is uniform from front to back implies that the occlusal planes of the maxilla and the mandible are parallel, as shown in Fig. **7**.

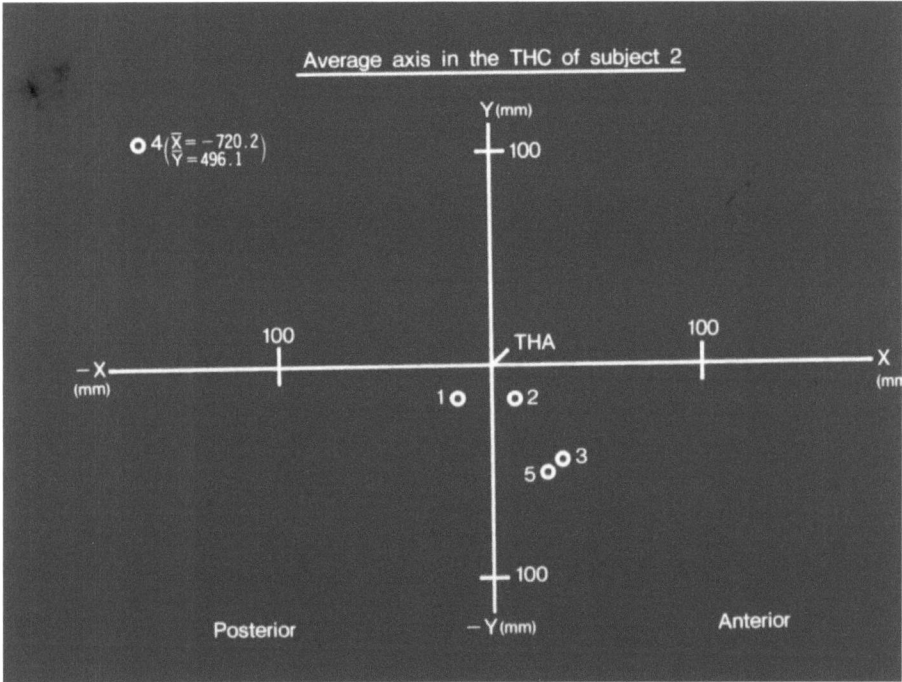

Figure 3: Average rotation centers of terminal hinge closure (THC) for subject 2.

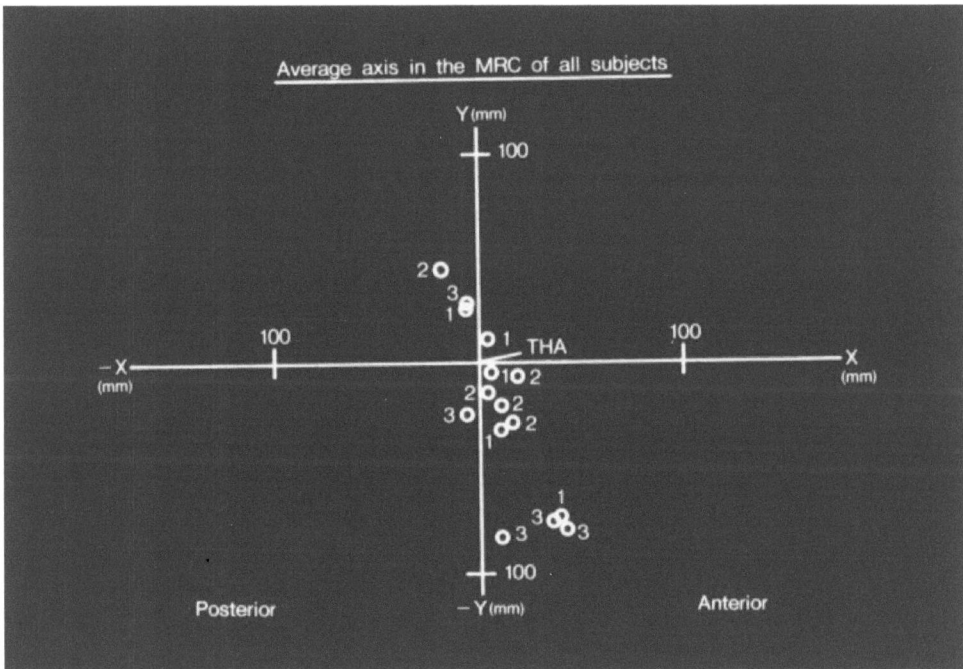

Figure 4: Average rotation centers of most retruded closure (MRC) for all subjects.

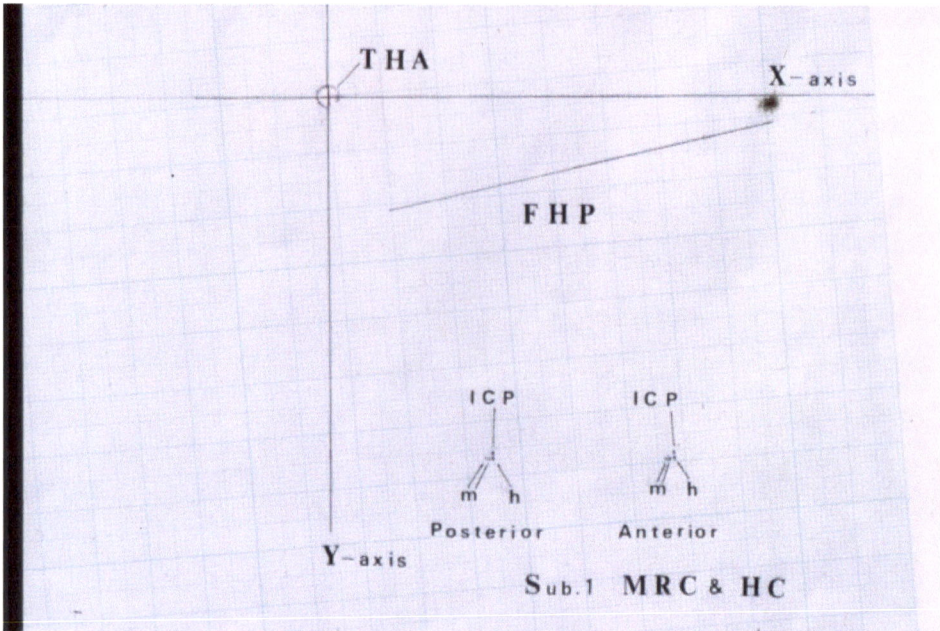

Figure 5: Sagittal plane recording of MRC and habitual closure (HC) for subject 1 using single sheet wax interocclusal record without metal foil *m* indicates MRC, *h* represents HC.

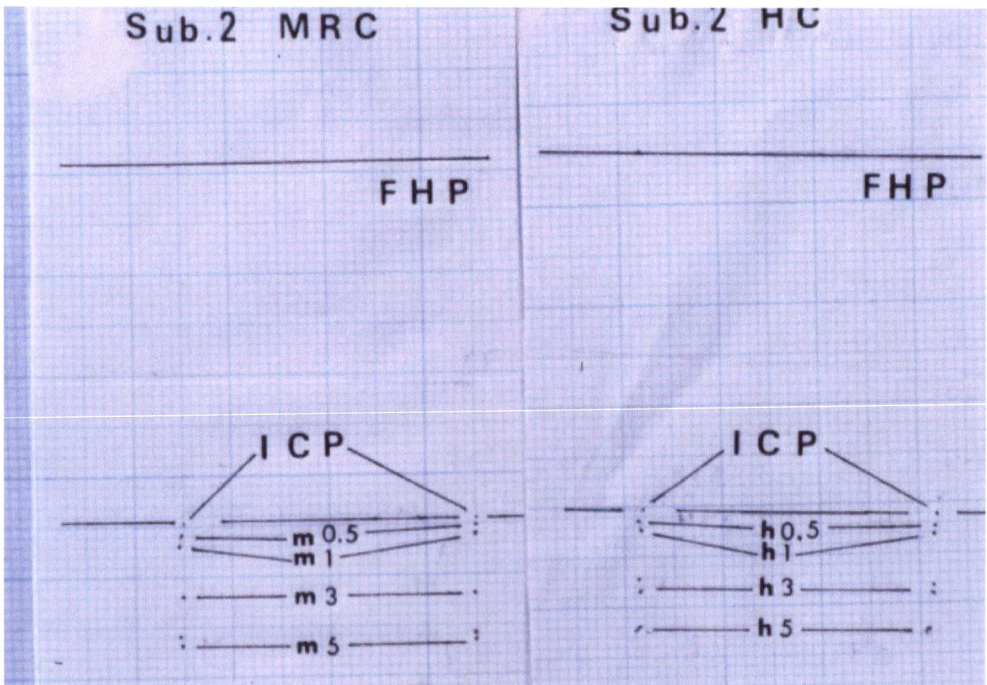

Figure 6: Frontal pane recordings of MRC and HC for subject 2.

Figs. **10** and **11** show the prototype. Torii compared the reproducibility of intraoral occlusal contact points in the ICP on articulators between a conventional articulator and the new articulator (prototype).

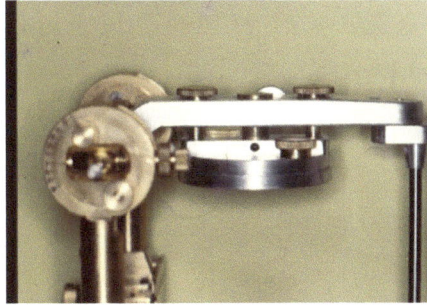

Figure 11: Prototype of an articulator with a vertical movable attachment.

The reproducibility of occlusal contact points in the ICP for the trial product was reported as statistically significantly superior to that of a conventional articulator (Fig. **12**) (Torii K, 1988). The reproducibility of occlusal contacts in the ICP (MCP or habitual contact position) is the most important for an articulator. An occlusal analysis and equilibration cannot be performed without a high degree of reproducibility in the MCP.

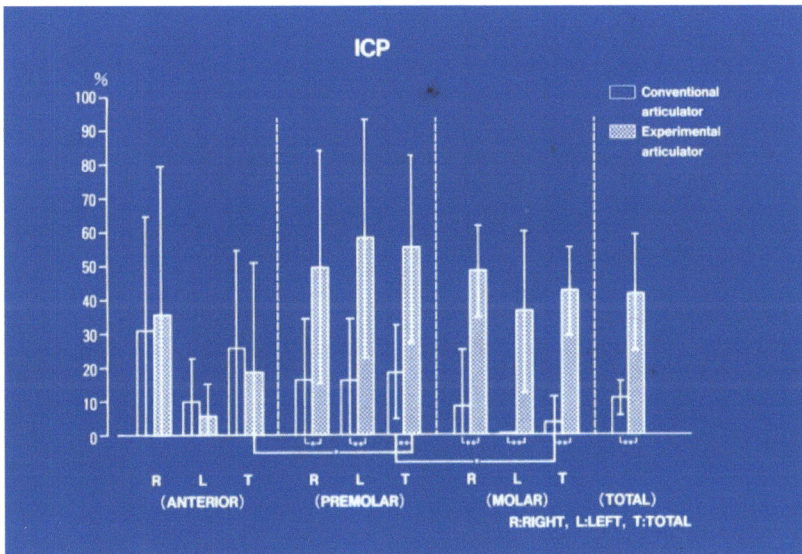

Figure 12: Comparison of the reproducibility of occlusal contacts in the ICP between conventional and experimental (prototype) articulators.

SUMMARY

The reproducibility of the MCP is required to be almost 100%, because the occlusal contacts of the MCP (that is the BPOP) cannot be confirmed directly in the mouth. Therefore, it is necessary to indirectly examine the occlusal contacts on an articulator that has a high reproducibility of the MCP.

REFERENCES

Alexander PC (1952). Movements of the condyle from rest position to initial contact and full occlusion. *J Am Dent Assoc* 1952;45:284-293.

Bennett NG (1958). A contribution to the study of the movements of the mandible. *J Prosthet Dent* 1958;8:41-51.

Brill N, Lammie GA, Osborne J, Perry H (1959). Mandibualr positions and mandibular movements: A review. *Brit Dent J* 1959;106:391-400.

Brown AH (1930). Movements of the mandible not provided for in present-day articulators. *J Am Dent Assoc* 1930;17:982-991.

Charles SW (1925). The normal movements of the mandible. *Brit Dent J* 1925;46:281-285.

Clapp GW (1952). There is no usable vertical opening axis in the mandible. *J Prosthet Dent* 1952;2:147-159.

Glickman I, Haddad AW, Martignoni M, Mehta N, Roeber FW, Clark RE (1974). Telemetric comparison of centric relation and centric occlusion reconstructions. *J Prosthet Dent* 1974;31:527-536.

Higley LB & Logan RA (1941). Roentgenographic interpretation of certain condyle and menton movements. *J Am Dent Assoc* 1941;28:779-785.

Luce CE (1889). The movements of the lower jaw. *Boston Med SJ* 1889;121:8-11.

McCollum BB (1939). Fundamentals involved in prescribing restorative dental remedies. *Dent Item of Int* 1939;61:522-535.

McCollum BB (1960). The mandibular hinge axisis and a method of locating it. *J Prosthet Dent* 1960;10:428-435.

Millstein PL, Kronman JH, Clark RE (1971). Determination of the accuracy of wax interocclusal registrations. *J Prosthet Dent* 1971;25:189-196.

Mitchell DL & Wilkie ND (1978). Articulators through the years. Part I. Up to 1940. *J Prosthet Dent* 1978;39:330-338.

Mitchell DL & Wilkie ND (1978). Articulator through years Part II. From 1940. *J Prosthet Dent* 1978;39:451-458.

Mohl ND (1991): Introduction to occlusion. In Mohl ND, Zarb GA, Calsson GE, Rugh JD, ed. *A textbook of occlusion.* Chicago: Qintessence, 1991:20.

Nevakari K (1956). A analysis of the mandibular movement from rest to occlusal position. *Acta Odontol Scand* 1956;14(Suppl 19):5-129.

Posselt U (1952). Studies in the mobility of the human mandible. *Acta Odontol Scand* 1952;(Suppl.10):20-150.

Shanahan TE & Leff A (1962). Mandibular and articulator movements Part III. The mandibular axis dilemma. *J Prosthet Dent* 1962;12:292-297.

The Academy of Prosthodontics (1999). *Glossary of Prosthodontic Terms.* 7-th ed. St. Louis: C.V. Mosby Co., 1999.

Thompson JR (1946). The rest position of the mandible and its significance to dental science. *J Am Dent Assoc* 1946;33:151-180.

Torii K (1989). Analysis of rotation centers of various mandibular closures. *J Prosthet Dent* 1989;61:285-291.

Ulrich J (1959). The human temporomandibular joint: Kinematics and action of the masticatory muscles. *J Prosthet Dent* 1959;9:399—406.

CHAPTER 6

Various Therapies Prior to Occlusal Equilibration

Abstract: There have been various therapies to relieve the symptoms of temporomandibular disorders. These therapies are required to relax the masticatory muscles and to precisely analyze, and equilibrate an occlusion in the muscular contact position (MCP).

Keywords: Masticatory muscles, occlusion, relaxation, appliance therapy, bite plane, occlusal splint, mandibular repositioning, muscle hyperactivity, anterior bite plate, electromyography, physical therapy, exercise therapy, biofeedback training, stress management, laser therapy, pharmacotherapy.

1. INTRODUCTION

Severe symptoms of temporomandibular disorders (TMDs) should be relieved prior to an occlusal analysis and occlusal equilibration, because the relationship between upper and lower jaws might be incorrectly deviated. Many therapies have been reported as having symptom-relieving action. These therapies are mainly classified into appliance therapy, physical therapy and pharmacotherapy.

2. APPLIANCE THERAPY

Occlusal splints or bite plates are widely used for the treatment of TMDs, even though their mechanism of action is unknown (Ramfjord SP & Ash MM, 1983, Okeson JP, 1981, McNeil C, 1990). Ramfjord and Ash described as follows: The terms bite plate and occlusal splint are often used interchangeably. Several different types of bite planes have been used in the treatment of structural and functional disturbances of the masticatory system. They have been used for the treatment of bruxism, TMJ-muscle pain dysfunction, trauma from occlusion, muscle tension headache, craniofacial pains, and various forms of arthritis involving the TMJ. Studies of the effectiveness of bite plane therapy generally support their effectiveness; predictability of treatment for functional disturbances involving the muscle and joints has been questioned. The effectiveness of stabilization bite planes has been questioned, usually as the basis for suggesting other or additional forms of therapy. Splints have been classified in a number of ways, but even the most elaborated classifications appear to have drawbacks for general acceptance. The use of the term stabilization to refer to bite planes that cover all the teeth (maxillary or mandibular) and thus splint the teeth together is reasonable, provided that the devices for "repositioning" and molar support only are not included and provided that term does not imply guiding the teeth into centric relation. Stabilization of the teeth should not be confused with stabilization of jaw position. The Hawley plate, Sved appliance, and Dessner bite plane have been referred to as relaxation-plane bite planes. Because their making is simple, the relaxation-plane bite plane have been advocated for the treatment of functional disturbances, including those disturbances considered to be related to mandibular "overclosure" with damage to the meniscus, condyle, and glenoid fossa, and for disturbances believed to be related compression of the Eustachian tube and the auriculotemporal and chorda tympani nerves. Although the latter was refuted, the relationship of mandibular overclosure to structural and/or functional disturbances remains controversial. The anterior bite plane is an effective appliance; however, relaxation-plane bite planes are not advocated- except for very short period of use- for the treatment of functional disturbances; clinical and animal studies indicate that the posterior teeth that are affected by a nonstabilization bite plane intrude into the alveolar process and cause the nonoccluding anterior teeth to extrude. The stabilization bite plane splint to be discussed here is sometimes referred to as the occlusal bite plane splint, the Michigan bite plane splint, or the Michigan occlusal splint. It has been reported that a higher percentage of patients improve with use of a full-coverage splint than other types, but it has also been suggested that all types of bite planes or occlusal splints are successful in 70-90% of treated patients. When isolation of the disturbing influences of occlusion is necessary- as with bruxism, trauma from occlusion, muscle hyperactivity (whether induced by peripheral and/or central influence), excessive abrasion of the teeth, so-called disk displacement, and some forms of arthritis- the use of a well-designed occlusal splint, and additional therapy if indicated, is effective treatment for most structural and functional disturbances of the masticatory system. By far, the best appliance for patients with dysfunctional symptoms is the occlusal splint, which covers all of the teeth in the mandible or in the maxilla. It is usually easier to fit the splint to maxilla than to the mandible. Regarding the mechanism of splint action, one simple explanation is that the bite plane causes a reduction in muscle hyperactivity. It may also provide the patient with a visible and physical reminder to reduce central influences that can result in muscle hyperactivity. Reducing muscle hyperactivity, increasing vertical dimension, and providing stable support for the mandible allow less stress to be placed on the joint structures. A flat plane-bite splint with freedom in splint centric allows the teeth to make contact with a stable supporting plane in an optimal position for comfort of the joints and muscles- both during swallowing and during the bracing of the teeth and mandible that appears to be required for lifting, pushing, and other types of physical activities. Several studies have demonstrated the effect of a splint on reducing muscle activity, the EMG silent period of masseter and temporalis muscles, and clinical symptoms. In addition, Ramfjord and Ash described as follows: There is evidence that mandibular repositioning takes place during effective bite plane therapy and that restriction of such movement may impede the relief of symptoms and even aggravate TMJ-muscle pain dysfunction. The evidence that an increased vertical dimension is a benefit of the bite plane is indirect and clinical. Muscle activity appears lesser at an increased vertical dimension and biting forces may be greater at an increased vertical dimension. An increased vertical dimension is not necessary for relief of symptoms; in some cases, however, relief of symptoms does not occur with splint therapy until the vertical dimension of the splint is increased beyond the point at which crepitus, clicking, tripping, or locking occurs. The role of possible protective reflexes involving the joint, teeth vertical dimension, and the necessity for a stable jaw position during certain physical activities is not clear. In summary, while other physiological and even psychological factors may be involved in effective splint therapy, the possible mechanism by which a bite plane influences the symptoms of TMJ-muscle pain dysfunction appears principally to be a reduction of muscle hyperactivity that is secondary to occlusal dysfunction. Muscle hyperactivity is reduced by the splint; the splint replaces disturbing occlusal influences with a nondisturbing occlusal platform, which allows the mandible to close into a stable position when bracing of the jaw is necessary during swallowing and physical exertion. The splint also allows optimal repositioning of the condyle, and it discourages bruxism, clenching, and abnormal bracing by removing the habitually used dysfunctional contact relations (Ramfjord S & Ash MM, 1983). Okeson *et al.* investigated the effects of occlusal splint which was provided simultaneous occlusal contact of all mandibular buccal cusp tips and incisal edges when the mandible was in the centric relation position. Adequate canine guidance was also provided to disarticulate all posterior teeth during eccentric movements. They reported as follows: Thirty-three TMD patients were treated for a 4-week period with the splint therapy. Fourteen muscle and joint regions were palpated before and after treatment, and observable pain scores were recorded. Maximal comfortable interincisal distance and maximal interincisal distance were recorded before and after treatment. The following results were obtained. 1. Out of the 33 patients, 28 showed significant improvement in observable pain score. The mean score was 4.4 ($p<.01$). 2. Out of the 33 patients, 27 showed increase in maximal comfortable interincisal distance. The mean increase in interincisal distance was 5.3 mm ($p<.01$). 3. Out of the 33 patients, 21 showed an increase in maximal mandibular opening; however, the increase of 1.7 mm was not statistically significant. 4. When the patients were divided into two groups according to the duration of symptoms, there was no significant difference between the group's symptoms or responses to treatment (Okeson JP *et al.*, 1982). On the other hand, Lundh *et al.* compared three treatment groups in sixty-three patients with an arthrographic diagnosis of disk displacement with reduction: (1) onlay to maintain disk-repositioning; (2): flat occlusal splint; (3): untreated controls. And they concluded as follows: The disk –repositioning onlays improved joint function and reduced joint and muscle pain when compared with the flat occlusal splint and with nontreatment. The signs and symptoms in the flat occlusal splint group were no different from those in the control group. It is concluded that disk-repositioning onlays are effective in reducing pain and dysfunction associated with disk displacement with reduction in patients in whom the disk can be maintained in a normal relationship to the condyle with the aid of such onlays. The symptoms, however, returned when the onlays were removed after 6 months; this raises the question of whether a permanent change in the intercuspal position is necessary for long-term success (Lundh H *et al.*, 1988). Ekberg *et al.* evaluated the short-term efficacy of a stabilization appliance in patients with TMD of arthrogeneous origin, using a randomized, controlled, and double-blind design. In the study, sixty patients were assigned to two equally sized groups: a treatment group given a stabilization appliance and a control group given a control appliance. And they concluded as follows: Improvement of overall subjective symptoms was reported in both groups but significantly more often in the treatment group than in the control group (P=0.006). Frequency of daily or constant pain showed a significant reduction in the treatment group (P=0.02) compared with the control group. The results of this short-term evaluation showed that both the stabilization appliance and control appliance had an effect on TMJ pain. It is improbable that the difference observed between the groups is due to chance alone (Ekberg E *et al.*, 1998). For using Michigan occlusal splint as described by Okeson (Okeson JP *et al.*, 1982), Ramfjord and Ash described as follows: The principal requirements are: (1) to provide for freedom from interference to any movement when the teeth are incontact with the splint; (2) to allow for closure of the mandible into a stable contact relation without interference; (3) to allow for a vertical dimension that can be adapted to readily; (4) to allow for lip seal if possible; (5) not to interfere with swallowing; (6) not to interfere with speaking; (7) not to interfere with buccal mucosa; and (8) to provide for the most favorable aesthetics under circumstances. The Michigan splint fits all the occlusal surfaces of the maxillary teeth and is held in place by the acrylic fitting into undercuts in the buccal interproximal dental areas. It is made up of heat-cured clear acrylic. The occlusal splint has a smooth surface, makes contact with the mandibular supporting cusps and has cuspid guidance. The cuspid guidance disoccludes supporting cusp contact almost as soon as lateral or protrusive mandibular movements are made. The reason for such disclusion is to eliminate as much feedback as possible from contacts away from the 'splint centric' (Ramfjord SP & Ash M, 1994). Dao *et al.*, evaluated the therapeutic efficacy of splints using a parallel, randomized, controlled and blind design for three groups: (1) passive control: full occlusal splint worn only 30 min. at each appointment; (2) active control: palatal splint worn 24 h/day; (3) treatment: full occlusal splint 24 h/day. And they reported that there were no significant differences between groups in any of the variables, and described that these data suggest that the gradual reduction in the intensity and unpleasantness of myofascial pain, as well as the improvement of quality of life during the trial, was non-specific and not related to the type of treatment (Dao TTT *et al.*, 1994). Al-Ani *et al.* analyzed 12 randomized control trials and compared stabilization splint therapy to: acupuncture, bite plates, biofeedback/stress management, visual feedback, relaxation, jaw exercises, non-occluding appliance and minimal/no treatment. They reported that there was no evidence of statistically significant difference in the effectiveness of stabilization splint therapy in reducing symptoms in patients with pain dysfunction syndrome compared with other active treatments, and there is a weak evidence to suggest that the use of stabilization splint for the treatment of pain dysfunction syndrome may be beneficial to reduce pain severity, at rest and palpation, when compared to no treatment (Al-Ani MZ *et al.*, 2004). Fricton concluded from the evidence-based review as follows: (1): Stabilization splints can reduce TMJ dysfunction pain compared to nonoccluding splints in those subjects with more severe TMJ dysfunction pain. There was no studies that demonstrated that splints work better in muscle pain, joint pain, or headache disorders, and in most studies, a mixed diagnosis of muscle and joint pain was present; (2): Stabilization splints in short term were equally effective in reducing TMJ dysfunction pain compared to physical medicine, behavioral medicine, and acupuncture treatment for TMJ dysfunction. However, the long-term effects of behavioral therapy may be better than splints in reducing symptoms in more severe patients where psychosocial problems may be present but definitive studies have not been done. In one study, stabilization appliance therapy was more effective than pharmacological treatment for headache pain suggesting more research is needed in headache patients; (3): Anterior positioning and soft splint have some evidence to suggest that they are effective in reducing TMD pain compared to placebo controls; (4): Anterior positioning splint are at least equal to or more effective in treating TMJ clicking and locking than stabilization splints; (5): Anterior bite planes have modest evidence of its efficacy for headaches and inconclusive evidence of effectiveness compared to a stabilization splint for TMJ dysfunction pain. There is a concern that partial coverage splints may contribute to tooth pain and/or occlusal changes and, thus, further study is needed before widespread use (Fricton J, 2006). Torii and Chiwata observed the changes of symptoms of TMDs and the mandibular positions using an anterior flat plane bite plate (Fig. **1**) (Torii K & Chiwata I, 2010). In their case report, the patient was diagnosed as having TMJ disc-displacement without reduction with arthralgia, and the symptoms completely disappeared in 2 weeks (Table **1**). McNeill also recommended an anterior bite plate for short-term use, because of the possibility of extrusion of teeth uncovered (McNeill C, 1990). Therefore, its use is recommended for 2 or 3 weeks.

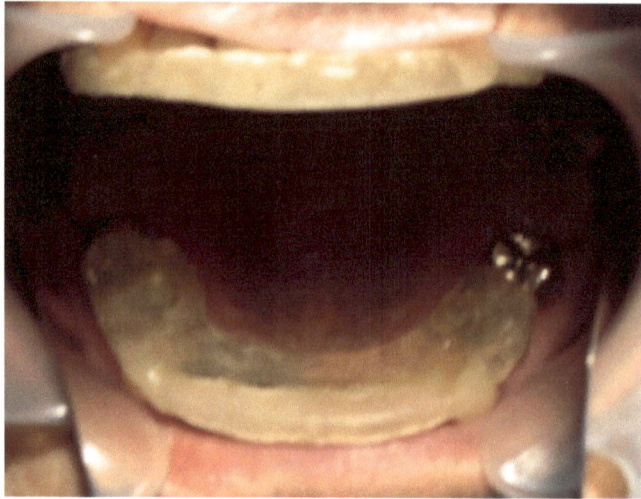

Figure 1: Anterior flat plane bite plate.

Table 1: Habitual occlusal position and bite plate-induced occlusal position and TMD symptoms on different days

NS	$H_1 B_1$	H_2				H_6	H_7			
S$\updownarrow$										
NS		B_2	$H_3 B_3$	$H_4 B_4$	$H_5 B_5$	B_6	B_7	$H_8 B_8$	$H_9 B_9$	$H_{10}B_{10}$
Days	1	3	6	9	12	15	25	33	50	110
VAS	6	3	2	2	0	0	0	0	0	0
Max.	40	42	42	42	42	45	45	45	45	45

NS: Not significant; S: Significant; Days: Days of visits; H_{1-10}: Habitual occlusal position on different days; B_{1-10}: Anterior bite plate-induced occlusal position on different days; VAS: Scores on a 10-point Visual Analogue Scale, where 0 denoted "no pain" and 10 denoted "worst pain".; Max.: Maximum unassisted opening (mm). Occlusal adjustment was performed on day 17.

Regarding the symptom relieving mechanism of occlusal splint, Manns *et al.* recorded the electromyographic (EMG) activities for various vertical occlusal dimensions and obtained minimal basal EMG activities at distances of 10-16 mm away from the occluded position (Manns A *et al.*, 1981). In their study, the vertical dimension was measured between the tip of the nose and chin-point. Therefore, the thickness of an anterior bite plate may be proper to be 7-8 mm. In addition, Manns *et al.* reported that elevator muscular activity during the use of an anterior block (like as anterior bite plate) was significantly lower than that during the use of three other posterior blocks and lower than that for an interocclusal position (Manns A *et al.*, 1993). In the case report of Torii and Chiwata (Torii K & Chiwata I 2010), muscular relaxation seemed to have occurred with the wearing of an anterior flat bite plate from the first visit until day 3, and this phenomenon might have been induced by a reduction in elevator muscle activity as a result of anterior bite raising. Consequently, the BPOP, which presents a physiological muscular position, was isolated from the combined HOP=BPOP position as a result of the muscular relaxation. The disappearance of the occlusal discrepancy between the HOP and the BPOP between day 6 and day 12 seemed to have been induced by the reprogramming of the voluntary jaw closing motor program arising from the central nervous system having learned a mandible position that reduces pain, and mandible closure at the BPOP shifted from the previous HOP. Kovaleski and De Boever reported that after the use of an occlusal bite plane splint for one month: (1) the mandible moves anteriorly and laterally on an occlusal bite plane splint where there is sufficient centric freedom built into the splint; (2) there is a decrease in TMJ-muscle symptoms provided anterior mandibular movement is not trapped by occlusal interferences, cuspid guidance, and/or incisal guidance on the splint; and (3) there is a decrease in the number of silent period elicited during tapping with the occlusal splint in the mouth. They used Michigan occlusal splint and reported the results as follows: The direction of the movement on the splint after 72 hours was most often towards the painful side and anteriorly directed. After 72 hours, six patients moved to side of painful joint, one to the opposite side, and one did not move. Out of the three patients with pain in both joints, one moved straight forward, and two moved laterally and anteriorly. After one month, the mandibles of the five patients stayed in the same position, as after 72 hours. In four patients, the mandibles moved a little more in the same direction. The patient who moved to the opposite side after 72 hours had moved to the side of the painful joint after one month. One patient moved back to the starting position. The extent of the mandibular movement varied from patient to patient and from one session to another, but never exceeded 3.5 ± 1.0 mm. After 72 hours, for nine patients, there was a mean anterolateral movement of 1.82 ± 0.93 mm. Two patients had a posterolateral mean movement of 2.6 ± 1.8 mm. After one month, for 10 patients, there was a mean anterolateral movement of 1.78 ± 0.97 mm. One patient had a posterolateral mean movement of 1.7 mm. With respect to symptoms, nine out of 11 patients reported pain and/or clicking relieved after 72 hours. All the patients were followed up to two months after the third treatment visit, and the occlusal adjustment was performed according to the technique advocated by Ramfjord and Ash. They all remained symptom free during a six-month follow-up (Kovaleski WC & De Boever J, 1975). Their results that the mandibular movement occurred after 72 hours of wearing occlusal splint agreed with the results of Torii and Chiwata in which the isolation of the BPOP and HOP occurred in three days. Fu *et al.* reported as follows: All subjects exhibited deviation (12subjects to the right and 8 subjects to the left) prior to bite plate therapy. After flat plane bite plate therapy, the mandibular position of all subjects shifted towards the labial frenum midline position. Based on the Binominal test, the shift was significant ($p<0.001$). Measurements on the Centric Check system showed a significant movement of both condyles in the antero-posterior plane as well as the vertical plane. There was also significant reduction in TMJ pain and clicking ($p<0.01$). The results support the hypothesis that the balanced position of the mandible is with frena aligned. When occlusal obstructions are eliminated, the mandible will drift to this position (Fu AS *et al.*, 2003). Sheikholeslam *et al.* myographically investigated the postural activity of the temporal and masseter muscles in thirty-one patients with signs and symptoms of functional disorders: before, during and after 3-6 months of occlusal splint therapy. They reported that the fluctuating signs and symptoms, as well as the postural activity of the temporals and masseter muscles were significantly reduced after treatment. Further, the coefficients of correlation within pairs of postural activity of the right and left muscles increased significantly. The results indicate that an occlusal splint can eliminate or diminish signs and symptoms of functional disorders and re-establish symmetric and reduced postural activity in the temporal and masseter muscles. They described as follows: The occlusal splint may be very valuable in the examination and treatment of patients with mandibular dysfunction. It is a simple device which can reduce signs and symptoms and established a more symmetric muscular rest activity. The splint also enhances procedure such as functional analysis and occlusal adjustment, and is a valuable tool which can be used for periods of several years, especially in patients where other forms of treatment are difficult to perform (Sheikholeslam A *et al.*, 1986). Clark *et al.*, performed an electromyographic study on twenty-five patients (18 women and 7 men) with TMDs. They used a portable EMG recording unit which is the compact EMG unit directly measured nocturnal activity of the masseter muscle for each patient. The EMG unit provided cumulative totals of electrical activity of the masseter muscle above 20 μV. The criterion of 20μV was selected to prevent recording of minor contraction of the masseter muscle that could not be defined as clenching or grinding. The EMG unit was activated at night after the patient had retired and it recorded unilateral activity of the masseter muscle during the hours of sleep. They reported as follows: Among all the patients, 17 had moderate symptoms and eight showed severe symptoms, according to the combined index of jaw dysfunction. Usually, the most frequent subjective complaint was a dull aching pain around the region of the TMJ. The most common (15 of 25 patients) clinical finding was that muscles of mastication were tender when examined. No one reported a history of dislocation of the TMJ, locking in a closed position, or severe symptoms of impaired function of the joints. Use of an occlusal splint had varied effects on nocturnal activity of the masseter muscle. Results were summarized as follows: Nocturnal EMG levels were significantly reduced during the use of splint in 13 (52%) of the 25 patients. Seven of the patients (28%) had no change and five (20%) had a significant increase in nocturnal EMG levels during the use of splints, 12 returned to pretreatment levels when the splint was removed. Effect of the splint on nocturnal EMG levels was compared according to severity of symptoms before treatment. Those with moderate symptoms were more likely to have a reduction in nocturnal EMG levels. Among the group with moderate symptoms, 64% had a significant decrease in nocturnal EMG level, whereas 25% of the group with severe symptoms showed a similar reduction. They described that splint was most likely to reduce nocturnal EMG levels in patients with least severe symptoms (Clark GT *et al.*, 1979). Carr *et al.* monitored the postural activities of jaw elevator and depressor muscles for healthy subjects (3 men and 3 women) using an occlusal splint. They reported that all postural muscle activities showed wide-ranging biological variation, but the activities induced by the splint tended to stabilize within 1 week, with decreased postural activities in the masseter and anterior temporalis muscles, and increased postural activities in the suprahyoid muscles (Carr AB *et al.*, 1991). Magnusson *et al.* reported a new type of splint as follows: This splint that covers the maxillary incisors, and has a point contact to the mandibular incisors, is said to reduce tooth clenching and grinding through "nociceptive trigeminal inhibition tension suppression system (NTI-tss)". And they reported that at the 6-month follow-up, 7 out of the remaining 10 subjects with NTI splints reported some (n=1) or significant (n=6) improvement, 2 reported no change and one reported impairment (Magnusson T, 2004). Jokstad *et al.* made comparison between two different splint designs for TMD therapy and reported as follows: No differences in treatment efficacy were noted between the Michigan and the NTI splint types when compared over 3 months (Jokstad A *et al.*, 2005). Schmitter *et al* performed a randomized clinical trials using two common splints for the treatment of patients with anterior disc displacement without reduction and reported as follows: As results of using centric splint (with bilateral occlusal contacts on the flat splint surface) and the distraction splint (occlusal contact are located predominantly in the posterior part of the splint), centric splint seem to be more effective than distraction splints. Therefore, before the surgical treatment of anterior disc displacement without reduction, centric splints should be used instead of distraction splints (Schmitter M, 2005). Williamson described repositioning splint therapy as follows: The response to treatment noted in the 464 patients indicates that repositioning splint therapy is an effective treatment modality for temporomandibular disorders (Williamson EH, 2005). On the other hand, Conti *et al.* performed a randomized clinical trial for the treatment of painful TMJ clicking with oral splints and reported that all of the subjects had a general improvement on the VAS, though subjects in the occlusal splint groups had better results that did subjects in the nonoocluding splint group (Conti PC, 2006). Wassell *et al.* described the treatment of TMDs with stabilizing splints or nonoccluding splint and reported that at one year, good response to TMD treatment in general practice had been maintained, but many subjects still had clicking TMJs (Wassell RW, 2006). Regarding the mechanism of the effect of splint on jaw muscles, Baad-Hasen *et al.* described that there were no effects of either NTI or OS (a standard flat occlusal splint) on clinical outcome measures. This short-term study indicated a strong inhibitory effect on EMG-activity in jaw closing muscles during sleep of the NTI, but not the OS (Baad-Hansen L, 2007). Alencar and Becker evaluated different occlusal splints associated with counseling and self-care in the management myofascial pain dysfunction and reported that all patients improved over time and all splint offered the benefit (Alencar F, Jr. & Becker A, 2009).

3. PHYSICAL THERAPY

These therapies are often used in combination with other therapy, mainly with occlusal splint therapy.

Exercise therapy includes various trainings, patient's self-training, small opening and closing training, active opening, or resistant opening *etc.* Maloney *et al.* compared the effectiveness of a passive jaw motion device, Therabite, and wooden tongue depressors, in patients with TMDs, who did not improve after manual manipulation of the mandible and flat bite plane therapy. The Therabite jaw motion rehabilitation device is a manually operated, patient controlled opening and closing device with an adjustable setting, set to the required vertical opening. The wooden tongue depressors (WTD) used for the study were standard wooden tongue depressors measuring approximately 1.25 mm in thickness and 14 mm in width. Two tongue depressors were placed bilaterally between the upper and lower teeth, and tongue depressors were added to gently force mouth opening and achieve a moderate stretch. Patients using the Therabite and the wooden tongue depressors were instructed to achieve and sustain a comfortable stretch of the jaw muscle. Patients were instructed to gently force their mouth open and hold the mouth open for one minute; then repeat this exercise three times in succession. This cycle of three openings was repeated five times per day. Patients presenting with maximum interincisal opening of less than 35 mm were chosen initially. The patients included in the study, 19 extracapsular (myogenous) and 24 intracapsular (arthrogenous), were allocated randomly to three treatment groups. The three groups were the Therabite group, wooden tongue depressor group, and control group. They reported as follows: For intracapsular group, there was a significant reduction in pain for subjects using the Therabite compared to subjects using wooden tongue depressors (p<0.013). There was no significant difference between the tongue depresoors and controls. Pain from pre-experimental period to the fourth week was reduced significantly in the subjects using the Therabite. For the subjects using the Therabite device, there was significant improvement in mouth opening after treatment (mean 27.2 to 35.4, t=-8.1, p<0.001). There was also significant improvement in the range of mouth opening for the WTD group (mean 29.3 to 32.0, t=-2.6, p<0.043). The control showed no significant change. For extracapsular group, Therabite produced significantly greater pain reduction than the WTD (p=0.05) and the control group (p=0.001). Pain was significantly reduced at the end of the study for subjects using the Therabite (mean 6.0 to 1.3, t=3.6, p=0.011). No significant change was observed for either the WTD or the control group. Increase in maximum mouth opening for patients in the Therabite group was significantly greater than wooden tongue depressors as well as controls. They summarized as follows: A passive jaw motion device (Therabite) is effective in increasing range of motion in both groups of TMD patients, joint (intracapsular) and muscle (extracapsular). Pain was relieved to a greater degree in the muscle group than the joint group (Maloney GE *et al.*, 2002). Magnusson and Syrén described the samples of jaw exercises (maximal jaw opening without resistance, jaw opening towards resistance, laterotrusion towards resistance and stretching) which were to be performed at least three times a day, and each treatment session should be at least 2-3 minutes. They compared the effect of appliance therapy and therapeutic jaw exercises in twenty-six patients fulfilled the strict inclusion criterias of TMD of mainly muscular origin. They summarized as follows: Half of the patients were assigned to receive treatment with an interocclusal appliance, the treatment being performed by a dentist. The other half was instructed to perform individualized therapeutic jaw exercises, and this treatment was managed by a dental assistant. The treatment result was evaluated after six months. The two treatments had a positive and equal effect upon both signs and symptoms of TMD. A further follow-up by questionnaire one to four years after the final clinical examination showed a lasting treatment result in most patients. Many patients, however, continued to perform jaw exercises and/or to wear their appliances. This indicates that these two treatments are mostly symptomatic and not causal. The conclusion of the present investigation is that therapeutic jaw exercises, managed by a dentist or a dental assistant, is a cost effective treatment with a prognosis comparable to a treatment with an interocclusal appliance and can thus be recommended as the first therapy of choice in patients with TMD of mainly muscular origin (Magnusson T & Syrén M, 1999).

Biofeedback training is to present a patient at his or her level of facial muscle tension using electromyographic recording. With auditory or visual feedback techniques, high-muscle tension is recognized by a fast rate of clicks, or by visual analogue/digital display, while a low-muscle tension is recognized by slow rate of clicks. The objective of biofeedback training in the patients with TMDs is to provide them with an insight into abnormal facial muscle activity, which include clenching and grinding of teeth habits. Principato and Barwell treated twenty-five patients using biofeedback in combination with relaxation program. They described as follows: Our program includes six to ten sessions of 40 minutes held at weekly intervals. Diaries are kept by each patient reflecting occurrence of symptoms and circumstances under which they occurred. These diaries provide further insight for the patients into the role that physical or emotional stress plays on the creation of their symptoms. In addition, these records allow for subjective appraisal of treatment response. The session begins when the patient is seated in a comfortable chair in a quiet and dimly lit room. A circumferential cutaneous frontalis lead is employed. The electromyographic levels are amplified and acoustically fed to the patient through earphones. Relaxation techniques are employed during the sessions. Such training provides the patient with an understanding of the existing levels of muscle tension and the influence of relaxation techniques on those levels of muscle tension. In this manner, the patient is provided objective evidence of his or her behavior-modifying capability. It is the long-term aim of these sessions to provide insight into facial habits and relaxation techniques capable of eliminating facial muscle tension and the symptoms of temporomandibular joint dysfunction on an ongoing basis. Office sessions are supplemented with one-hour relaxation programs at home on a daily basis. They reported that the number of sessions provided for each patient was six, and 70-80% of TMD symptoms were relieved, and objective comparison of frontalis muscle tension levels between the first and sixth sessions demonstrated significant reduction in maximum and minimum recorded levels (Principato JJ & Barwell DR, 1978). On the other hand, Turk *et al.* evaluated the efficacy of two treatment modalities: intraoral appliances (IA) and biofeedback, separately and in combination (BF/SM). The first study of their studies compared intraoral appliance treatment (n=30), a combination of biofeedback and stress management (n=30), and a 6-weeks waiting list control condition group (n=20) for TMD patients. The procedures were described as follows: *Interocclusal appliance treatment.* Patients received a full-arh interocclusal appliance. The appliance was a flat heat-cured acrylic resin splint and was constructed on the maxillary or mandibular arch. Patients were instructed to wear the appliance at all times for the first 6 weeks of treatment, except during eating and oral hygiene. To control the frequency of professional contact, these patients were seen weekly by a dentist for 6 weeks, as in the BF/SM treatment condition described next. During each session, patients were instructed in oral habits, such as avoiding chewing gum and eating soft foods. *Biofeedback/stress management treatment.* Patients assigned to the BF/SM condition were seen for 6 weekly 1-hour sessions by a psychologist trained in biofeedback-assisted relaxation procedures and SM. The specific BF procedures used were as follows: (1) 4 mm Ag/AgCl surface electrodes were taped bilaterally over the masseter muscle; (2) to ensure that electrodes were in the same position each session, a plastic template showing the position of the electrodes was made for each patient; (3) computer controlled auditory tone and pulsating feedback directly proportionate to masseter muscle tension levels was used; and (4) each BF session began with a no-feedback resting baseline period of 5 minutes, during which time patients were instructed to relax their jaw muscles to best of their ability, followed by 20 minutes of BF, and concluding with a 5 minutes no-feedback period. In addition to BF during each treatment session, BF/SM patients were also provided with SM therapy that included (1) didactic education regarding the association between stress, increased muscle tension, and pain; (2) training in several cognitive coping skills to control pain, for example, attention diversion; and (3) homework assignments to help patients practice relaxation skills without the BF instrumentation, as well as techniques to identify stressful situations in their natural environments and ways to deal more effectively with these sources of stress. *Waiting list control group (WL).* Patients assigned to the WL group received the same pretreatment assessment procedures as the IA and BF/SM groups. At the time of the pretreatment evaluation, WL patients were informed that there was a waiting list for treatment and were scheduled for a second appointment 6 weeks later. At their second appointment, these patients received an assessment procedure identical to the first. The patients then were provided with either IA or BF/SM treatment, but were not included in any of the analyses that compared treatment outcome between the IA and BF/SM conditions. In their second study, the effect of a treatment protocol that combined the IA and BF/SM treatments was evaluated. They reported as follows: The appliance treatment was more effective than the biofeedback and stress-management treatment in reducing pain after treatment, but at a 6-month follow-up the appliance treatment group significantly relapsed, especially in depression, whereas the biofeedback and stress-management treatment group maintained improvements on both pain and depression and continued to improve. In addition, the combination of appliance and biofeedback-stress-management was more effective than either of the single treatment alone, particularly in pain reduction, at 6-month follow-up (Turk DC *et al.*, 1993).

Laser therapy as a treatment for TMDs was reported by Hansson (Hansson TL, 1989). According to Hansson, therapeutic experience and preliminary results of experimental studies suggest a role for laser therapy with its antiphlogistic, antiedematous, and stimulative effects on cellular metabolism, with secondary effects on pain. Since distinction between myogenous and arthrogenous pain is possible, the clinical application of laser technology to the elimination of an intra-articular inflammatory process should be considered. Hansson performed the pilot therapeutic trial for five TMD patients and reported as follows: *Osteoarthrosis.* Pain as reported by the patient disappeared within the first days of treatment. An accompanying increase of mouth opening was registered (2 and 5 mm, respectively) and the TMJ crepitation sounds were dramatically reduced during the time of laser application. *Postoperative TMJ pain.* Patients reported that pain started to diminish after the initial applications. The mouth opening increased (2 and 26 mm, respectively). The crepitation sounds were reduced both in magnitude and in their position of the mandibular movement. Both of these observations were noted by the author. The sounds were located at the end of mouth opening after the laser treatment compared with their pretreatment locations. Stable mandibular function remained during the 1-year follow-up period when occlusal stability was achieved and maintained. *Anterior disk displacement.* Pain disappeared after the initial sessions of application. The mouth opening increased by 10 mm during the 5 days of application. Hansson described as follows: Laser treatment is not proposed as an alternative to conventional reversible treatment of conditions with arthrogenous pain. However, it seems possible to reduce the time for healing of such conditions. The rapid reduction of inflammation by the infrared laser may contribute to a stable occlusion and symmetrical muscle function that in turn, will effectively influence the reparative processes. A possible sequence of treatment for arthrogenous craniomandibular pain as result of this preliminary report may be hypothesized accordingly: (1) Reversible splint-induced mandibular stabilization; (2) Inflared laser application, five sessions of 3 minutes each at 700 Hz; (3) Continued mandibular stabilization (1 month);

Permanent stabilization with wearing of the splint until rehabilitation is completed (Hansson TL, 1989). In the author's clinical experience, the following case was very difficult to relief the symptoms of TMDs: A 50 –year-old man presented with complains of his left TMJ pain and limitation of opening mouth. The maximum unassisted opening was 26 mm. The patient reported pain on the left TMJ during the opening. A stabilizing occlusal splint was fabricated and the patient worn it. Since no change in mouth opening and pain during 14 days, a cool laser light exposure was chosen for the patient (Fig. **2**). The mouth opening increased by 20 mm after the initial session, but pain persisted. Therefore, the combination of splint and laser exposure was continued during 3 months until pain subsided.

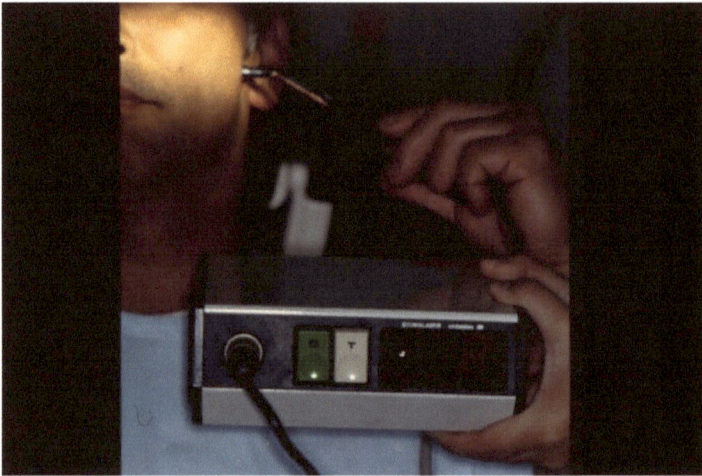

Figure 2: Infrared laser exposure.

Nelson and Ash evaluated the effectiveness of a moist heating pad as an adjunct to occlusal bite plane splint therapy in 27 patients between the ages of 20 and 70 years, with TMJ/muscle dysfunction. They described as follows: As an adjunct to outlined conventional TMJ therapy, the experimental patient group (19) applied moist heat with a 110/115-volt automatic moist heating unit, capable of heating to 160°F. The treatment temperature of the unit was patient modulated through a manual (on/off) in-line control switch. Depressing the switch (on) yielded a temperature increase, and releasing the switch (off) deactivated the unit. The cloth covering of the unit was described as drawing atmospheric humidity and required no specific moistening procedures. Instructions were given to the experimental group for unilateral application or bilateral/cervical application to include the primary areas of discomfort. In general, the patients were instructed to recline if possible and to apply the fomentation unit for 20 minutes, two-three times a day at temperature tolerance. Discontinuation of the heat treatment was recommended in the event of increased dysfunction or inflammatory tissue reaction, however, none was encountered. The remaining eight patients served as controls. The difference between the within group mean differences for mean analog scale values, when comparing experimental and control groups, was interpreted as demonstrating that the use the moist heating pad was an effective adjunct to bite splint therapy for TMJ/muscle dysfunction. The mean change within the heating pad group reflected a 34.7% reduction in symptoms compared to a 3.75% reduction in the control group on the analog scale. The percentage difference in mean differences of the two groups was 92% in favor of the heating pad group. They concluded that the use of a moist heating pad is an effective adjunct to bite plane splint therapy (Nelson SJ & Ash MM, 1988).

Kirk and Calabrese investigated the effect of physical therapy on internal derangement of TMJ in sixty-eight patients. In their investigation, patients were classified into five categories of disc displacement. Assignment was based on the time of occurrence of the opening clicking: opening reciprocal clicks that occurred between 0 and 15 mm interincisal opening, grade I; 15 to 30 mm, grade II; 30mm to end of condylar translation, grade III. Treatment modalities for disc displacement consisted of techniques described by Rocabado and were administered by a physical therapist. These included manual joint distraction; extensive exercise program; and others for the TMJ and cervical/thoracic regions. Pain control techniques included ultrasound, phonophoresis, transcutaneous electrical nerve stimulation (TENS), high-voltage galvanic stimulation, acustimulation, ice, moistheat, massage, and joint rest. No attempts were made to categorize pain control results based on the mode of therapy. Evaluation of pain relief was based on subjective patient information. All patients were initially treated once or twice a week for a 3- to 6-week period by the physical therapist. Treatment was considered successful if clicks were eliminated, range of motion was unimpeded by abnormal disc dysfunction, and there was a significant decrease or relief of pain. These are some of the same criteria for the success suggested by the American Association of Oral and Maxillofacial Surgeons. Posttreatment follow-up of pain control and joint function was performed by the surgeon. Clinical examination and telephone interviews were used for this assessment. Patients in whom clicking returned during the follow-up period were not considered as successfully treated with physical therapy. Posttreatment evaluation was continued for 3 years. If physical therapy was not successful after this initial treatment period, the patient was referred back to the oral and maxillofacial surgeon for further evaluation. Attempts to diagnose the degree of intra-articular pathology were then undertaken. Examination was focused on diagnosis of disc dysfunction, deformity, and internal derangement. Surgery was subsequently performed on 22 patients in whom physical therapy failed. Surgical findings were correlated with the degree of dysfunction and postulates formed as to the reason for failure. They reported as follows: Twenty-eight out of 51 patients (53%) with suspected mild- to moderate-stage disc displacements were successfully treated with physical therapy only. Seven out of 19 patients with grade I clicks required simple occlusal appliances (Sved type) to assure successful disc recapture, and nine out of 32 patients with grade II clicks did so. A success rate of 86% (44/51) was achieved in these two groups when appliances-assissted physical therapy was included. These appliances were worn for 1 to 3 months in all cases and then discontinued. Follow-up continued while appliances were worn and until disc dysfunction was improved and maintained without wearing the appliance. Physical therapy was not early nearly as successful in the patients with grade III clicking, locking, or clicking on mediolateral excursion. No patient in the last group was helped by physical therapy. Likewise, only four of 19 grade III joints were successfully managed. Three of these four were diagnosed as chronically hypermobile joints. Hypermobility was defined as vertical incisal opening >50 to 55 mm, with radiographic evidence of condylar excursion well beyond the articulating eminence, and history of two or more episodes of dislocation. Only four of 17 patients with anteriorly displaced nonreducing discs were successfully treated. Three of the four patients successfully treated were judged to be in an acute phase without prior subjective history of internal derangement. After further evaluation, it was felt that these three patients were locked because of trauma. One patient was felt to have myositis from a dental injection. These three patients, and the three patients with chronic hypermobility, were removed from the study. This resulted in a total of 28 of 30 joints (93%) in the grade III and locked categories that did not respond to physical therapy with or without bite appliances. The findings from the comparison of the grade of the disc displacement with the duration of subjective perception of displacement suggest that the majority of patients with grade I clicks were symptomatic for 1 year or less. Patients with grade II clicks showed the widest distribution of duration of symptoms, with awareness anywhere from 6 months to more than 5 years. No patient with grade III click could recall symptoms of less than 2 years duration. More than 50% of this sample noted symptoms present for 5 years or longer. Patients with joint locking appeared to have had the symptom for 1 year or less. Only three patients could be identified as having had no prior symptoms or signs of clicking. The majority of these patients had noted symptoms of clicking for many years. None of the patients received prescribed analgesics during treatment. Fifty-two of the 87 joints in this group of patients were rendered pain-free or exhibited marked reduction in pain. Forty-two out of 52 patients (81%) were in the grade I and grade II categories. Only ten out of 36 patients (28%) in the grade III locked categories experienced pain relief or a decrease in pain with physical therapy. It should be noted that in some cases, pain was much decreased but the click remained. They summarized as follows: A success rate of 86% was achieved in patients with early- to mid-opening and late- to mid-closing clicks of TMJ. Approximately one third of these patients required short-term occlusal bite appliances to assist in their management. A success rate of 7% was achieved in patients with late-opening and late-closing clicks. No patients with clicking on mediolateral movement were successfully managed with physical therapy. Likewise, patients with nonreducing anteriorly displaced discs of TMJ did not respond well to physical therapy. Pain management was evaluated separately and showed subjective improvement in 82% of patients with mild to moderate disc dysfunction and pain. Only 29% of patients with late-opening clicking or locked joints experienced pain relief. Twenty-two patients who did not respond favorably to physical therapy underwent surgical procedures. Findings in these patients offer suggestions about why nonsurgical therapy is not successful in certain cases (Kirk W & Calabrese D, 1989). Truelove *et al.* reported that all patients improved over time, and traditional splint therapy offered no benefit over the SS (a soft vinyl splint) therapy. Neither splint therapy provided a greater benefit than self-care treatment without splint therapy (Truelove E *et al.*, 2006).

4. PHARMACOTHERAPY

Pharmacotherapy of TMD includes analgesics, nonsteroidal anti-inflammatory drugs, corticosteroids, muscle relaxant, antianxiety agents, and antidepressants (McNeill C, 1990). The nonopiate analgesics are effective for mild to moderate pain, and Aspirin is the prototype. Opioid narcotics are the most useful in controlling acute severe pain but are less effective in controlling chronic pain. Nonsteroidal anti-inflammatory drugs (NSAID) are effective against mild to moderate inflammatory conditions and postoperative pain. The indications include treatment of synovitis, capsulitis, myositis, and as an alternative to narcotic analgesics for the treatment of more severe pain. Corticosteroids are not commonly prescribed for systemic use in the treatment of inflammation associated with TMD. Muscle relaxants are prescribed to help prevent the increased muscle activity associated with TMD. Anti-anxiety agents (Benzodiazepines) have proven useful in decreasing nocturnal masseter muscle conditions. The tricyclic antidepressants are beneficial in doses as low as 10 mg in the treatment of muscle contraction headache and musculoskeletal pain, and in doses of 25 to 100 mg, are beneficial in the treatment of chronic orofacial pain and various oral dysesthesias, including glossodynia and idiopathic oral burning (McNeill C, 1990). Regarding differential diagnosis of orofacial pain using oral medications, Ram *et al.* described as follows: Chronic orofacial pain is a rapidly evolving and challenging field that deals with the management of pain originating from neurogenic, osseous, muscular, or vascular structures of the head and neck. The challenge lies in the accurate diagnosis of orofacial pain conditions, which may be difficult to differentiate in many clinical situations. As pain cannot be "seen" or precisely located or its intensity measured with any device, clinicians must rely heavily on the patient's own description of type, duration and location of pain, and thus, history plays a crucial role in diagnosis. Advances in neuroscience, pharmacology, and pain management have made medications as one of the primary therapeutic modalities in the management of pain including orofacial pain conditions. Despite this, these medications will not help patients if the origin and nature of pain is not accurately diagnosed. Hence, diagnosis is critical for the successful management of orofacial pain conditions. Experience and knowledge of practice in pain management have led clinicians to devise several clinical diagnostic tests using medications in various forms (topical, oral, injections, intravenous infusions) to differentiate certain orofacial pain disorders where the nature of pain is unclear and the presentation of pain is multiple sites. Although the diagnostic tests are not 100 percent accurate, they are very effective in many clinical scenarios, especially in orofacial pain conditions. Topical medications such as anesthetics and anti-inflammatories, oral medications such as anti-inflammatory drugs and skeletal muscle relaxants, injections such as local anesthetics and corticosteroids, and vapocoolant sprays are some examples of the modalities used by clinicians to manage orofacial pain conditions. These medications may also be used for diagnostic tests to aid in accurate diagnosis of some orofacial pain conditions. In addition, there are special cases where medications such as triptans, carbamazepine and indomethacin may be used as diagnostic tests to confirm diagnosis of migraines, neuralgias, or stabbing headaches, respectively. Based on the concept of using medications to predict which treatment would be best for certain pain conditions or to aid in better diagnosis, diagnostic intravenous infusions of lidocaine, morphine, and ketamine have been studied to test the response to adjuvant analgesics and oral dextromethorphan. Paradoxically, taking the patients off their current medications can be of diagnostic significance in conditions like medication overuse headache and serotonin selective reuptake inhibitor-induced clenching. They described the use of medications in detail as follows: The orofacial pain conditions for which NSAIDs are often prescribed initially are arthralgia, capsulitis, arthritis, myofascial pain, and a locked TMJ. The commonly used NSADs are ibuprofen and nabumetone. The recommended oral dosage for ibuprofen is 600 mg qid or 800 mg tid, not to exceed 3200 mg/day. The recommended dosage for nabumetone is PO 500mg to 750 mg or tid, up to 1500 to 2000 mg/day. In suspected cases of tension-type headaches, NSAIDs such as ibuprofen or naproxen sodium (220 mg in divided doses up to maximum of 660 mg per day) may be used as the first line of choice. The drugs used for relief of chronic regional musculoskeletal pain include carisoprodol, chlorzoxazone, cyclobenzaprine hydrochloride, metaxalone, methocarbamol and orphenadrine citrate. These medications are generally used only in acute clinical proven spasm and not for the long term. When acute muscle spasm is suspected, cyclobenzaprine hydrochloride (5 mg to 10 mg bid) is often administered for short periods of time to see if the jaw pain decreases and mobility increases. In the cases of limited mouth opening, the vapocoolant spray and stretch is used diagnostically to differentiate between limited mouth opening due to muscle spasm or extracapsular restriction. An increase in mouth opening on using the spray and stretch is indicative of limited mouth opening secondary to trismus (Ram S *et al.*, 2006).

SUMMARY

Appliance therapy is the first choice to relief severe symptoms, such like pain and limited mouth opening. A stabilizing occlusal splint is suited for long-term use and an anterior flat plane bite plate is for short-term use. However, an anterior flat plane bite plate is necessary for occlusal analysis and equilibration (see chapter 7).

REFERENCES

Al-Ani MZ, Davies GJ, Gray RJM, Sloan P, Glenny AM (2004). Stabilization splint therapy for temporomandibular pain dysfunction syndrome (Review). *Cochrane Database Syst Rev* 2004;CD002778.

Alencar F, Jr. & Becker A (2009). Evaluation of different occlusal splints and counseling in the management of myofascial pain dysfunction. *J Oral Rehabil* 2009;36:79-85.

Baad-Hansen L, Jadidi F, Castrillon E, Thomsen PB, Svensson P (2007). Effect of a nociceptive trigeminal inhibitory splint on electomyographic activity in jaw closing muscles during sleep. *J Oral Rehabil* 2007;34:105-111.

Carr AB, Christensen LV, Donegan SJ, Ziebert GJ (1991). Postural contractile activities of human jaw muscles following use of an occlusal splint. *J Oral Rehabil* 1991;18:185-191.

Clark GT, Beemsterboer PL, Solberg WK, Rugh JD (1979). Nocturnal electromyographic evaluation of myofascial pain dysfunction in patients undergoing occlusal splint therapy. *J Am Dent Assoc* 1979;99:607-611.

Conti PC, dos Santos CN, Kogawa EM, de Castro Ferreira Conti AC, de Araujo C dos R (2006). The treatment of painful temporomandibular joint clicking with oral splints: a randomized clinical trial. *J Am Dent Assoc* 2006;137:1099-1107.

Dao TTT, Lavigne GJ, Charbonneau A, Feine JS, Lund JP (1994). The efficacy of oral splint in the treatment of myofascial pain of the jaw muscles: a controlled clinical trial. *Pain* 1994;56:85-94.

Ekberg EW, Sabet ME, Petersson A, Nilner M (1998). Occlusal appliance therapy in a short-term perspective in patients with temporomandibualr disorders correlated to condyle position. *Int J Prosthodont* 1998;11:263-268.

Fu AS, Mehta NR, Forgione AG, Al-Badawi EA, Zawawi KH (2003). Maxillomandibular relationship in TMD patients before and after short-term flat plane bite plate therapy. *J Craniomandib Pract* 2003;21:172-179.

Fricton J (2006). Current evidence providing clarity in management of temporomandibular disorders: Summary of a systemic review of randomized clinical trials for intra-oral appliances and occlusal therapies. *J Evid Base Dent Pract* 2006;6:48-52.

Hansson TL (1989). Infrared laser in the treatment of craniomandibular disorders, arthrogenous pain. *J Prosthet Dent* 1989;61:614-617.

Jokstad A, Mo A, Krogstad BS (2005). Clinical comparison between two different splint designs for temporomandibular disorder therapy. *Acta Odontol Scand* 2005;63:218-226.

Kirk WS & Calabrese DK (1989). Clinical evaluation of physical therapy in the management of internal derangement of the temporomandibular joint. *J Oral Maxillofac Surg* 1989;47:113-119.

Kovaleski WC & De Boever J (1975). Influence of occlusal splints on jaw position and musculature in patients with temporomandibualr joint dysfunction. *J Prosthet Dent* 1975;33:321-327.

Lundh H, Westesson PL, Jisander S, Eriksson L (1988). Disk-repositioning onlays in the treatment of temporomandibular joint disk displacement: Comparison with a flat occlusal splint and with no treatment. *Oral Surg Oral Med Oral Pathol* 1988;66:155-62.

Maloney GE, Mehta N, Forgione AG, Zawawi KH, Al-Badawi EA, Driscoll SE (2002). Effect of a passive jaw motion device on pain and range of motion in TMD patients not responding to flat plane intraoral appliances. *J Craniomandib Pract* 2002;20:55-65.

McNeill C (1990). Management, In:*Craniomandibular disorders, Guidelines for evaluation, diagnosis, and management,* McNeill, pp.(33-47), Quintessence, ISBN:0-86715-227-3, Chicago.

Magnusson T & Syrén M (1999). Therapeutic jaw exercises and interocclusal appliance therapy. *Swed Dent J* 1999; 23:27-37.

Magnusson T, Adiels AM, Nilsson HL, Helkimo M (2004). Treatment effect on signs and symptoms of temporomandibular disorders—comparison between stabilization splint and new type of splint (NTI). A pilot study. *Swed Dent J* 2004;28:11-20.

Manns A, Miralles R, Guerrero F (1981). The changes in electrical activity of the postural muscles of the mandible upon varying the vertical dimension. *J Prosthet Dent* 1981;45:438-445.

Manns A, Rocabado M, Cadenasso P, Miralles R, Cumsille MA (1993). The immediate effect of the variation of anteroposterior laterotrusive contact on the elevator EMG activity. *J Craniomandib Pract* 1993;11:184-191.

Nelson SJ & Ash MM (1988). An evaluation of a moist heating pad for the treatment of TMJ/muscle pain dysfunction. *J Craniomandib Pract* 1988;6:335-359.

Okeson JP (1981). Etiology and treatment of occlusal pathosis associated facial pain. *J Prosthet Dent* 1981;45:199-204.

Okeson JP, Kemper JT, Moody PM (1982). A study of the use of occlusion splint in the treatment of acute and chronic patients with craniomandibular disorders. *J Prosthet Dent* 1982;48:708-712.

Principato JJ & Barwell DR (1978). Biofeedback training and relaxation exercises for treatment of temporomandibular joint dysfunction. *Otolaryngology* 1978;86:766-769

Ramfjord SP & Ash MM (1983). Diagnosis and treatment, In: *Occlusion* (Third Edition), Ramfjord & Ash, pp. (359-379), Saunders, Philadelphia.

Ramfjord SP & Ash MM (1994). Reflections on the Michigan occlusal splint. *J Oral Rehabil* 1994;21:491-500.

Ram S, Kumar SKS, Clark GT (2006). Using oral medications, infusions and injections for differential diagnosis of orofacial pain. *CDA J* 2006;34;645-654.

Sheikholeslam A, Holmgren K, Riise C (1986). A clinical and electromyographic study of the long-term effects of an occlusal splint on the temporal and masseter muscles in patients with functional disorders and nocturnal bruxism. *J Oral Rehabil* 1986;13:137-145.

Schmitter M, Zahran M, Duc JM, Henschel V, Rammelsberg P (2005). Conservative therapy in patients with anterior disc displacement without reduction using 2 common splints: a randomized clinical trial. *J Oral Maxillofac Surg* 2005;63:1295-1303.

Turk DC, Zaki HS, Rudy TE (1993). Effects of intraoral appliance and biofeedback/stress management alone and in combination in treating pain and depression in patients with temporomandibular disorders. *J Prosthet Dent* 1993;70:158-164.

Toii K & Chiwata I (2010). A case report of the symptom-relieving action of an anterior flat plane bite plate for temporomandibular disorder. *The open Dentistry J* 2010;4:218-222. ISSN 1874-2106.

Truelove E, Huggins KH, Mancl L, Dworkin SF (2006). The efficacy of traditional, low-cost and nonsplint therapies for temporomandibular disorder: a randomized controlled trial. *J Am Dent Assoc* 2006;137:1099-1107.

Wassell RW, Adams N, Kelly PJ (2006). The treatment of temporomandibular disorders with stabilizing splints in general dental practice: one-year foolow-up. *J Am Dent Assoc* 2006;137:1089-1098.

Williamson EH (2005). Temporomandibular dysfunction and repositioning splint therapy. *Prog Orthod* 2005;6:206-213.

Send Orders for Reprints to reprints@benthamscience.net

CHAPTER 7

Occlusal Equilibration in the Muscular Contact Position

Abstract: Occlusal equilibration in the muscular contact position (MCP) is required to obtain bilateral occlusal contact in the MCP. It is essential to equilibrate an occlusion on dental casts mounted on an articulator with bite plate-induced occlusal position wax record (BPOP record).

Keywords: Occlusal equilibration, bite plate-induced occlusal position, articulator, anterior flat plane bite plate, limited mouth opening, intercondylar distance, wax record, mandibular position analyzer, premature occlusal contact, occlusal tape, muscular conditioning, occlusal adjustment, muscle tenderness, occlusal restoration, prosthodontics, orthodontics, wedge shaped space.

1. INTRODUCTION

Occlusal equilibration in the muscular contact position (MCP) is very difficult to obtain in the mouth, because the MCP is very unstable. This is because avoiding movement in the deflective premature occlusal contact tends to shift the MCP to the more stable ICP (intercuspal position). Therefore, occlusal analysis and equilibration in the MCP should be performed on casts mounted on an articulator with a bite plate- induced occlusal position (BPOP) wax record.

2. PROCEDURE OF OCCLUSAL ANALYSIS AND EQUILIBRATION

An anterior flat plane bite plate should be fabricated directly in the mouth using a self- curing acrylic resin material; the vertical dimension should be sufficient to produce a 1- mm jaw separation in the second molars. The plate should cover the upper six anterior teeth and both first premolar teeth. The occlusal surface of the plate should be flat and perpendicular to the mandibular incisors to allow free movement in all directions (Figs. **1** and **2**). To fabricate an anterior flat plane bite plate, acrylic resin is lightly pressed against the upper anterior teeth and the first premolar teeth and a template of celluloid is placed over the resin. The patient is asked to lightly close his or her mouth until the lower anterior teeth contact the template and slide the teeth freely until the acrylic has set.

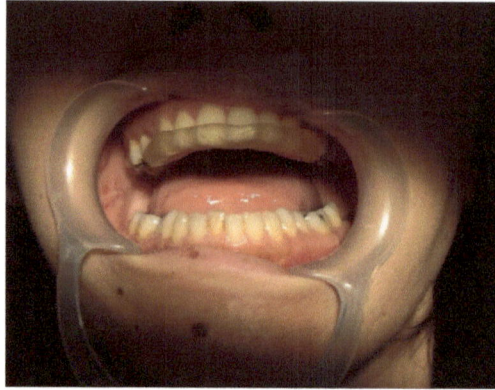

Figure 1: Anterior flat plane bite plate.

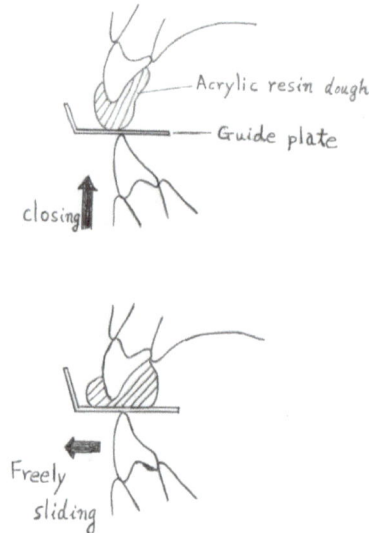

Figure 2: Fabrication of an anterior flat plane bite plate.

If the patient has limited mouth opening, the patient should wear the bite plate while tapping and sliding his or her lower anterior teeth against the plate for five minutes, then open the mouth as widely as possible. This procedure should be repeated for 10 to 20 minutes until the limitation disappears. Once the patient is able to open his mouth widely without experiencing any pain, he/she should proceed to the next step. If limited mouth opening does not resolve during the first visit, the patient should be instructed to wear the plate all day and to continue the exercise with bite plate for a week. During that period, if free opening is not obtained, other therapies such as pharmacotherapy or physical therapy, may be necessary to achieve easy mouth opening. Once the patient can freely open his mouth, he should proceed to the next step.

Two sets of upper and lower dental casts are made. Three habitual occlusal position (HOP) records are obtained using a vinyl polysiloxane bite registration material in an upright position without headrest support. Three bite plate-induced occlusal position (BPOP) records are then obtained using the same material as that used to record the HOP. After wearing the bite plate for 5 minutes, during which the patient continues to tap and slide his lower anterior teeth against the plate, then plate is removed and a vinyl polysiloxane bite registration material is applied with a syringe over the occlusal surfaces. The patient is asked to close his mouth until the point where the teeth come into contact with each other and hold that position until the material is set (approximately one minute). Then, three BPOP wax records are obtained using a wax registration material (Bite wafer, Kerr USA., Romulus, MI, USA) using the same procedure described above. The anterior part of the wafer is then cut off and softened at 60°C for 7-8 seconds. After muscular conditioning using the bite plate, the softened wafer is placed on the premolars and molars of the maxilla on both sides. The patient is instructed to bite the wafer gently, without biting through the wafer. The record is trimmed of excess wax, cooled with an air spray, and removed from the mouth (Figs. **3** and **4**).

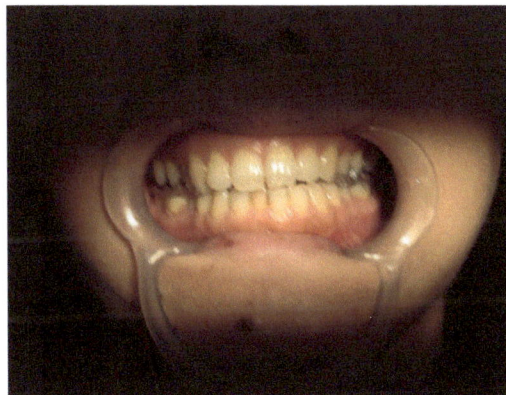

Figure 3: Registration of the MCP.

The BPOP wax record is trimmed of excess wax before removal.

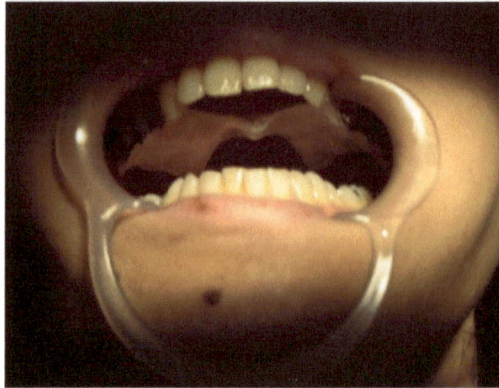

Figure 4: Removing the BPOP wax record.

The **w**ax record is cooled with an air spray.

Next, the intercondylar distance is measured using a caliper. The distance between the condylar point and the lower incisal point in the occluded position is also measured using a caliper (Figs. **5a** and **6a**).

The intercondylar distance of an articulator is set to the same value as that of the patient (Fig. **5b**).

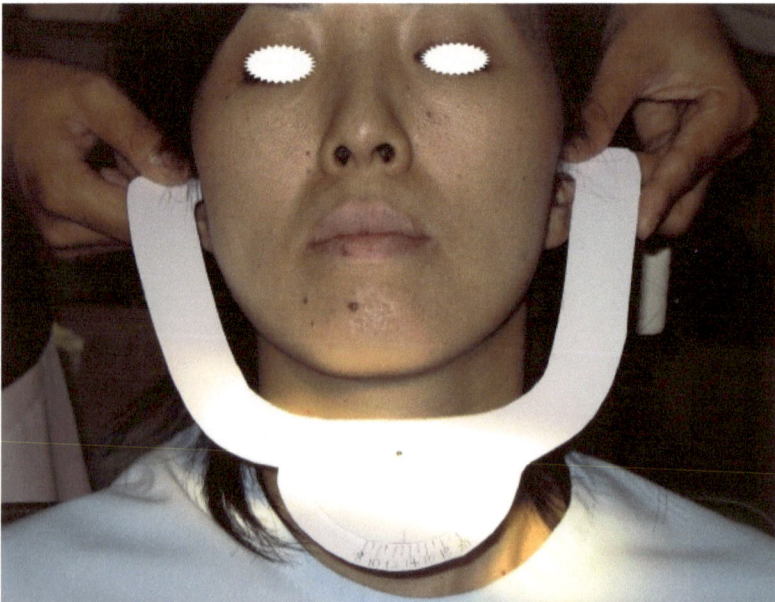

Figure 5a: Measuring intercondylar distance.

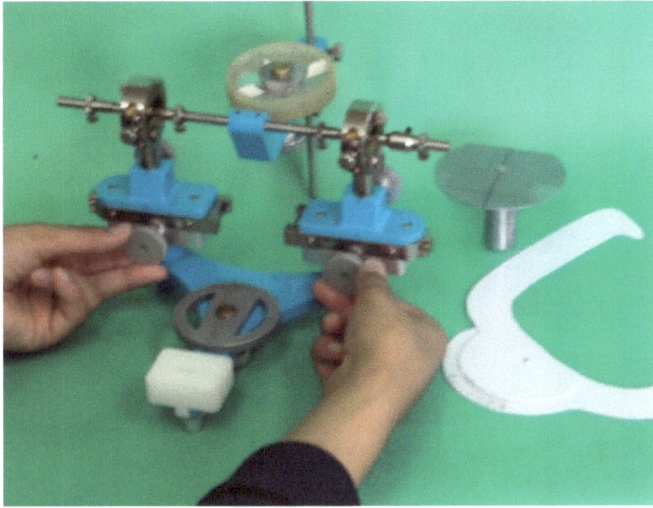

Figure 5b: Setting the intercondylar distance of an articulator.

The zero graduation on both sides of the scale indicates 13 cm of intercondylar distance (the distance is between the outsides of both condylar spheres). Therefore, when the intercondylar distance of the patient is 12 cm, the scale should be reduced medially by 5 mm on each side. The articulator is then inverted and placed on the plastering stand and the mandibular cast table is attached onto the upper mounting plate. A midline is marked on the surface of the lower cast base. With a white pencil, an incisal point is marked on the midline of the table at a point that is the same distance from the condylar ball of the articulator as that of the patient (Fig. **6a** and **b**).

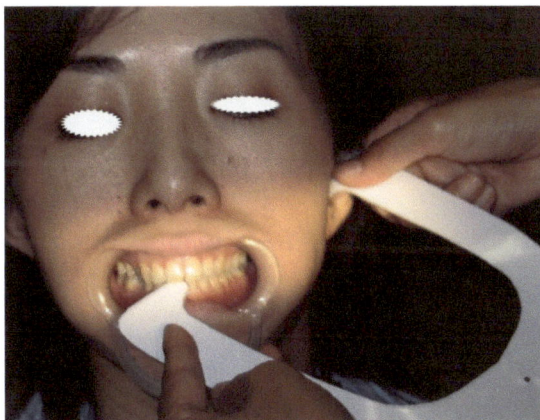

Figure 6a: Measuring the distance between the incisal point and condylar point.

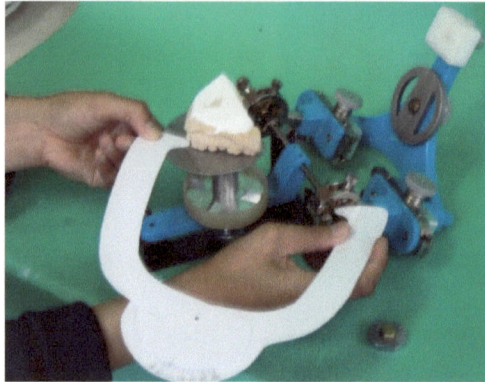

Figure 6b: Locating the lower cast.

The lower cast is located at the same position in the patient and attached to the lower mounting plate using plaster. After the plaster has set, the table is exchanged with a maxillary retentive nut, and the plastering rim is fitted to the upper mounting plate. A BPOP wax record is fitted between the two casts, and the base of the upper cast is covered with a sheet of wrapping film (Fig. **7**).

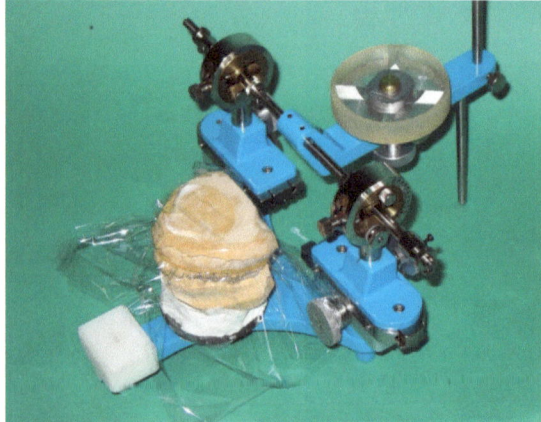

Figure 7: Covering the upper cast with wrapping film to separate the attaching plaster.

The first layer of plaster is poured into the mounting rim so that the height of the bulk of plaster is kept at a distance of 2 cm from the base of the upper cast (Fig. **8**). After the first poured plaster has set, a second layer of plaster is added on top of the first plaster. Then, the articulator is closed. Once the plaster has set, the film is removed, and then an α –cyanoacrylate adhesive material is injected between the upper cast and the mounting plaster (Fig. **9**). This mounting method prevents the dimensional change that occurs during setting of the plaster and subsequent inaccuracy of the articulated casts.

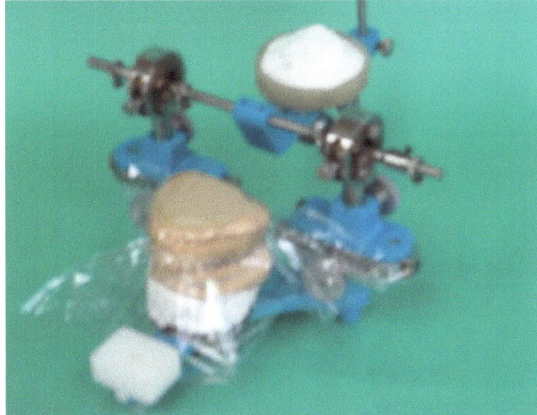

Figure 8: Mounting of the upper cast to the upper member in two steps.

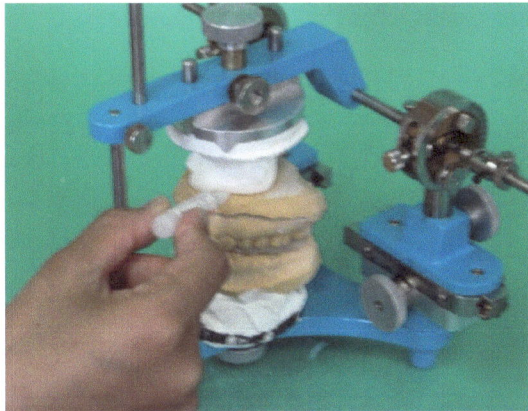

Figure 9: Accurate mounting of the casts.

The upper cast and the mounting plaster are attached with an adhesive material.

Consistency of the three BPOP wax records should be confirmed using a split cast method.

Both condylar rods are exchanged with the analyzing rods, and the recording discs are inserted into the condylar shaft. The vinyl polysiloxane HOP record is inserted between the upper and lower casts, and the positions are marked on the discs with colored occlusal paper (Fig. **10**).

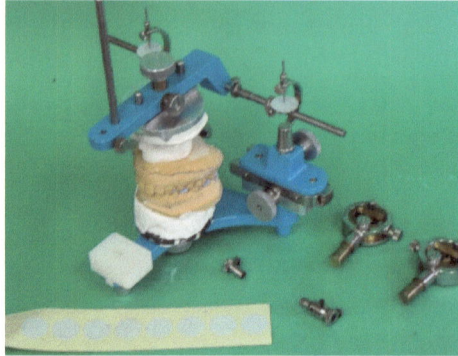

Figure 10: Mandibular position analyzer.

The articulator is used as the mandibular position analyzer.

In the same manner, the BPOP is recorded on the discs using different colored occlusal paper. The difference between the HOP and BPOP should be noted in addition to the direction from the BPOP to the HOP.

After recording the BPOP and HOP, the analyzing rods are changed back to the condylar rods, and the wax BPOP record is inserted between the two casts, and all adjustable settings are fixed. The BPOP wax record is removed and the vertical movable attachment screw is loosened. The upper cast is then moved downward until tooth contact is made (Fig. **11**).

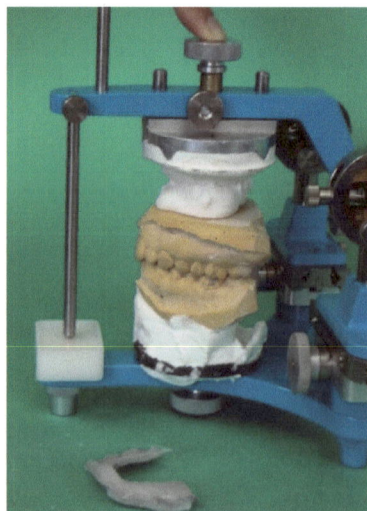

Figure 11: Vertical movement of an articulator.

After removing the BPOP wax record, the upper cast moves downward until the teeth come into contact.

The premature occlusal contact is located on the articulator by pulling an occlusal tape (Occlusion foil; Coltène/Whaledent, D-89122 Langenau, Germany) (Fig. **12**).

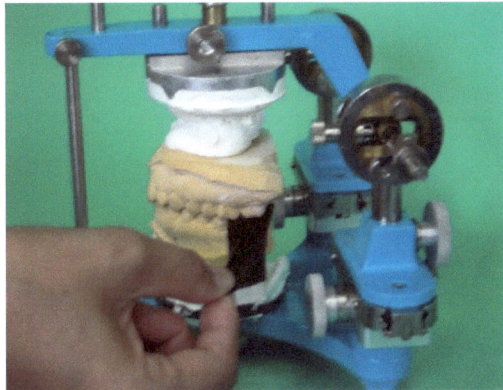

Figure 12: Detection of premature contact.

Premature contact is detected by pulling an occlusal tape.

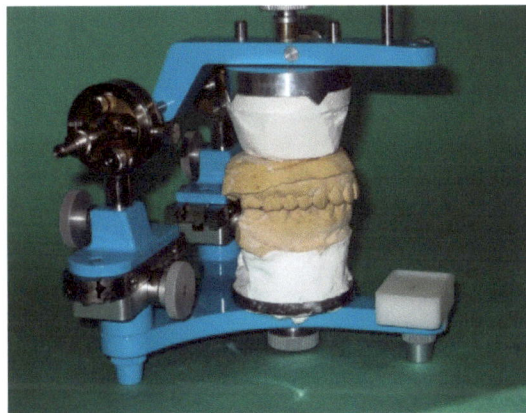

Figure 13: Hinge movement of articulator.

The premature contact is removed using a small pear shaped carbide bur (MG77MF HP 023, Hager & Meisinger GmbH, Dusseldorf, Germany) with a slow speed handpiece. The ground spot is marked with a colored pencil. The incisal pin is then removed from the upper member of the articulator, which is then closed to make the teeth contact, because when the mandible elevates vertically from the rest position to the tooth contact position, the condyle is pressed against the disc and rotates around the axis approximately located in the condyle (Figs. **13-15**). Then, the next premature contact is detected by pulling an occlusal tape and is removed with the bur. The ground spot is marked with a different colored pencil from the previously used one.

After removing the premature contact, the incisal pin is removed from the articulator to allow hinge movement.

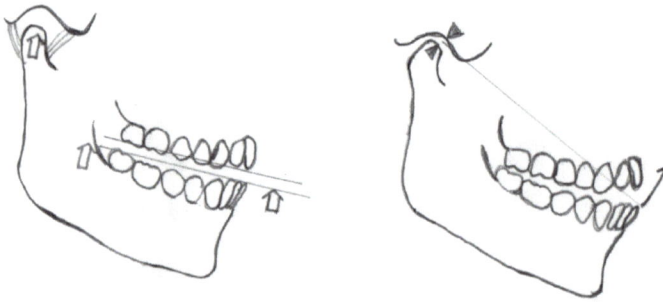

Figure 14: The shift from bodily movement to hinge movement

When the mandible vertically elevates, it rotates around the rotation center positioned approximately in the condyle.

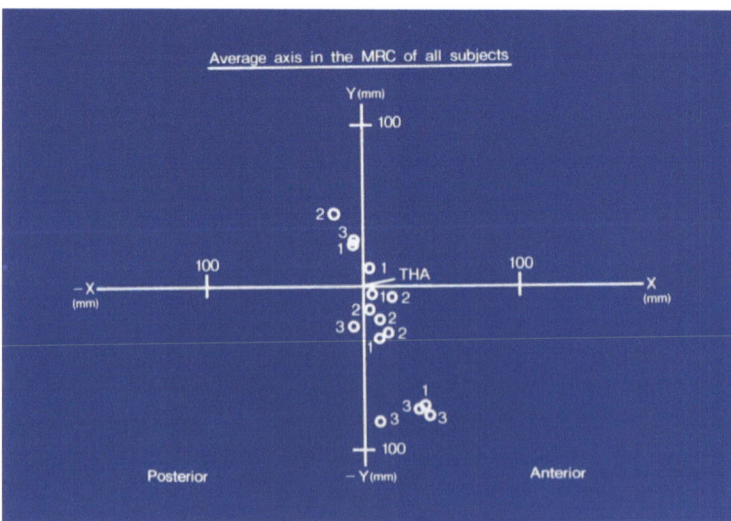

Figure 15: The average rotation center of the MRC for all subjects.

The most retruded closure (MRC) was achieved with the subject was in a supine position.

The mandible was retruded as far as possible by the subject's own effort (Torii K, 1989).

The patient is seated in an upright position. Then the anterior flat plane bite plate is worn in the mouth. After muscular conditioning by tapping and sliding the lower anterior teeth against the plate for 5 minutes, the plate is removed from the mouth and an occlusal tape is located in the mouth with a Millar ribbon holder (Buffalo Dental Manufacturing Co., Inc. Brooklyn, New York, USA). The patient is then asked to close the jaw until the teeth come into contact and to hold that position. The premature occlusal contact is confirmed by pulling the tape laterally. The premature contact should be compared with the contact marked on the articulator. The occlusal contact coincident with the one located on the articulator is selected as the true premature contact. The patient is reclined and the premature contact is removed using a high speed handpiece and a diamond point of similar size and shape to the previous carbide bur (Diamond point FG, 265R, SHOFU Inc. Kyoto, Japan). The patient is then raised to an upright position, and the bite plate is worn in the mouth. After the muscular conditioning, an occlusal tape is again inserted into the mouth and the next premature contact is detected. If the next contact is located at the same position as that on the articulator, the articulator can be regarded as precisely reproducing the BPOP (MCP) and the articulator can be reliably used in the following steps during future appointments. When the next premature contact is ground, impressions of the upper and lower jaw are obtained along with the BPOP wax record as previously described. The upper and lower casts are fabricated and mounted on the articulator with the BPOP wax record for the next appointment. Continued occlusal adjustments are made in the mouth by referring to the marked points on the casts mounted on the articulator and repeating from steps (5) to (7). In one session, only two or three contacts should be removed because adaptation to the new occlusion may take place between sessions. In this way, a stable occlusal position can be established with minimal grinding. The occlusal adjustment is completed by confirming the occlusal contacts on the premolar and molar teeth on both sides of the casts mounted on the articulator and in the mouth. If a large amount of grinding teeth is required to equilibrate the occlusion, some restorations may be needed. In some cases, the premature contact appears on the anterior teeth; therefore, the examination should always be performed on the full arch of dentition.

Torii and Chiwata reported that in their study on occlusal adjustment, the number of visits varied between 2 and 34 (mean, 11.0 ± 6.0) and the treatment period ranged between 0.2 and 7.0 (mean, 2.8 ± 2.1 months) months. The bite plate wearing period ranged from 1 and 21 (mean, 9.6 ± 6.7) days, and between 1 and 13 (mean, 4.7 ± 3.5) sessions of occlusal adjustment were conducted (Torii K & Chiwata I, 2010).

We now report the case of a patient in whom occlusal adjustment therapy was applied. A 39-year-old woman was presented with chief complaints of sleep bruxism, hypersensitivity of the lower left second molar and severe right-sided headache. She was diagnosed with myofascial pain. Occlusal analysis was performed with dental models mounted on an articulator, and a discrepancy between the HOP and BPOP was identified in association with deviation of the mandible to the right side (Figs. **16-20**).

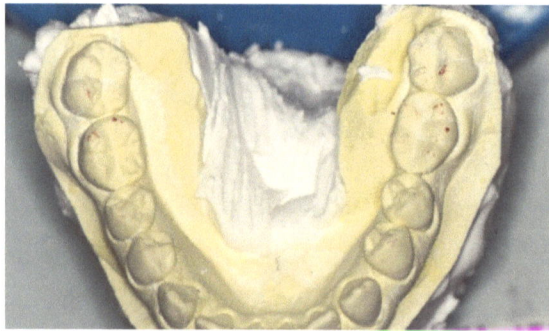

Figure 16: Recorded premature contacts on the lower cast.

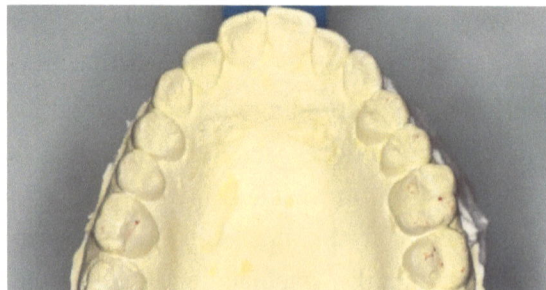

Figure 17: Recorded premature contacts on the upper cast.

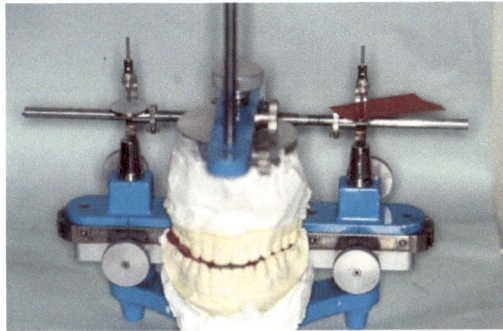

Figure 18: Analyzing of mandibular position.

The BPOP (MCP) was marked on the mandibular position analyzer.

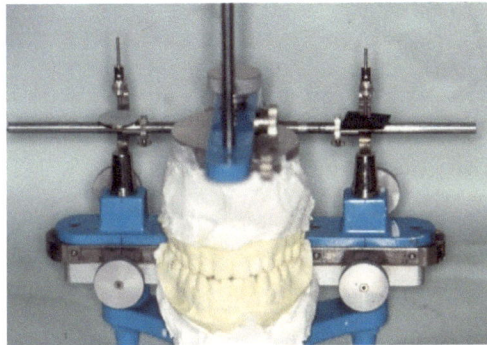

Figure 19: Recording HOP.

The HOP was marked in a different color from BPOP on the analyzer.

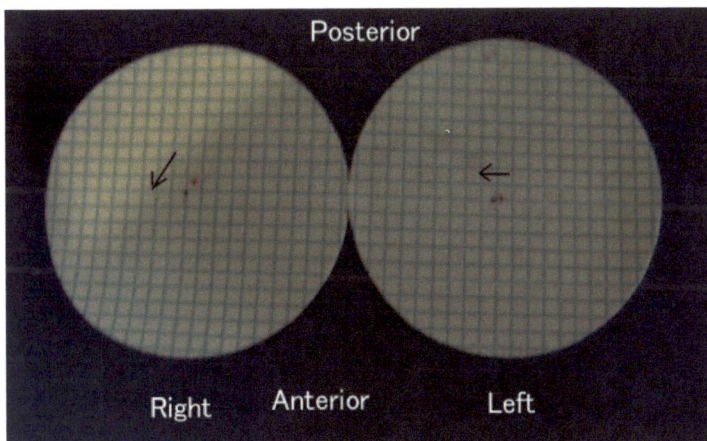

Figure 20: The recorded occlusal discrepancy between HOP and BPOP.

The mandibular position was shifted to the right from the BPOP (MCP).

Occlusal adjustments in the BPOP were then performed for this patient h (Fig. **21**). The headache scores were recorded before and after treatment on a 10-point Visual Analog Scale (VAS), where 0 denoted "no pain" and 10 denoted "worst pain". She had been diagnosed as having migraine.

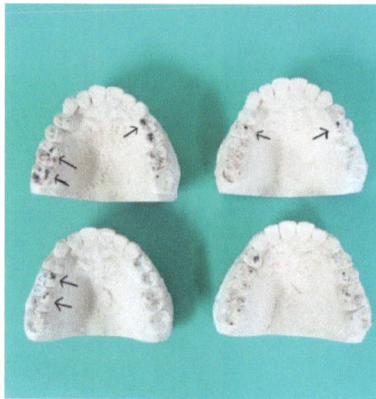

Figure 21: Premature contacts on different sessions.

The occlusal adjustments described above were performed step by step in four sittings with intervals of one week between each sitting (Fig. **21**). Meanwhile, the adhesion bridge was also reconstructed because of the lack of occlusal contact of the right first premolar. The occlusal adjustment was completed after confirming the occlusal contacts on the bilateral premolar and molar teeth on the casts mounted on the articulator and in the mouth (Figs. **22** and **23**).

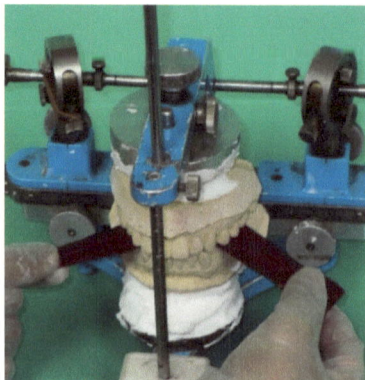

Figure 22: Confirmation of occlusal contacts on the articulator.

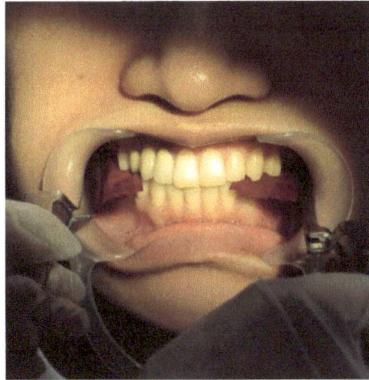

Figure 23: Confirmation of occlusal contacts in the mouth.

The VAS score for headache decreased from 10 to 6 following treatment. However, the migraine attacks persisted during the treatment period. The patient reported resolution of the fatigue and pain in the jaw and neck every morning. In addition, she never developed facial swelling again. The frequency of bruxism was decreased. On palpation, there was no tenderness of the masticatory muscles, except the right lateral pterygoid muscle.

Another case was that of a 25-year-old woman who presented with a chief complaint of limited mouth opening and pain in the right temple, the neck and shoulder. She reported that she was often having pain in the left temporomandibular joint (TMJ) region and limited mouth opening. The patient's medical history was not remarkable. With regard to occlusion, no midline deviation was evident, and the vertical and horizontal overlaps were very small (Fig. **24**).

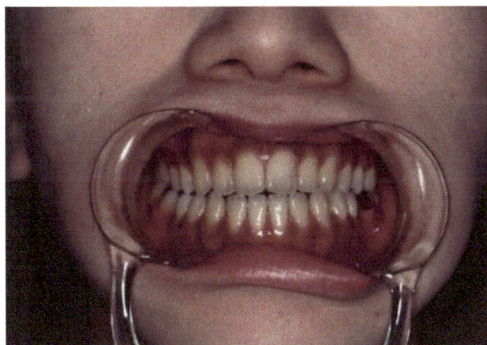

Figure 24: The Occlusal relationship in the habitual occlusal position.

The patient's maximum unassisted opening was 28 mm. She reported tenderness on palpation of the left TMJ and tenderness of the right anterior temporalis, the right platysma and sternocleidomastoideus, and the left external and medial pterygoideus muscles. The opening path deviated to the left side. She reported the stuffy ear on the left side in addition to eye symptoms (flashing at the bottom of the eyes). She was diagnosed as having myofascial pain with limited opening based on the Research Diagnostic Criteria for TMD (RDC/TMD) (Dworkin SF & LeResche L, 1992). An occlusal splint was fabricated and inserted in her mouth (Fig. **25**).

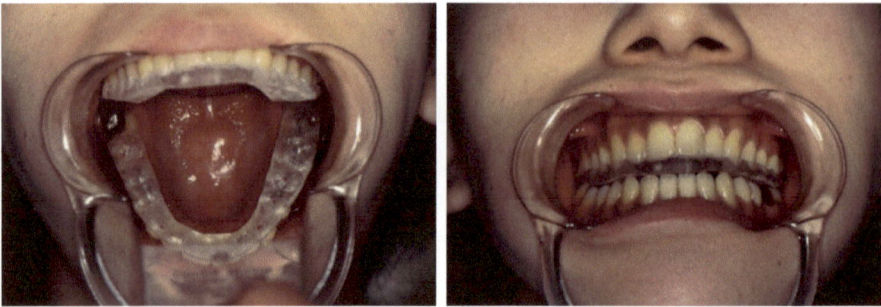

Figure 25: A flat plane occlusal splint.

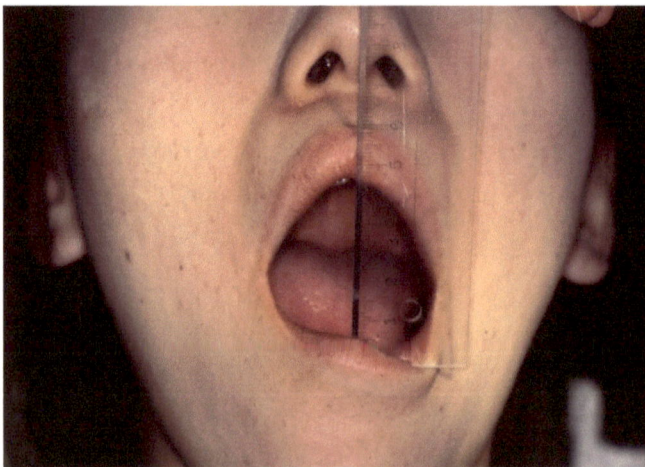

Figure 26: Unassisted opening of the mouth after wearing an occlusal splint for one week.

After wearing the occlusal splint for one week, the patient's maximum unassisted opening increased to 45 mm (Fig. **26**). After wearing the splint for two weeks, the tenderness of all muscles except for the left external and medial pterygoideus and the sternocleidomastoideus was relieved. BPOP wax records were then obtained, and the dental casts were mounted on an articulator with the BPOP wax record. The condylar posts were replaced by analyzing rods and an occlusal analysis was performed (Fig. **27**). The analysis showed that the HOP was deviated anterolaterally on the left side and posteromedially on the right side (Fig. **28**). The analyzing rods were again replaced by the condylar rods. After the BPOP wax record was removed, the upper mounting plate was moved down until the teeth came into contact (Fig. **29**).

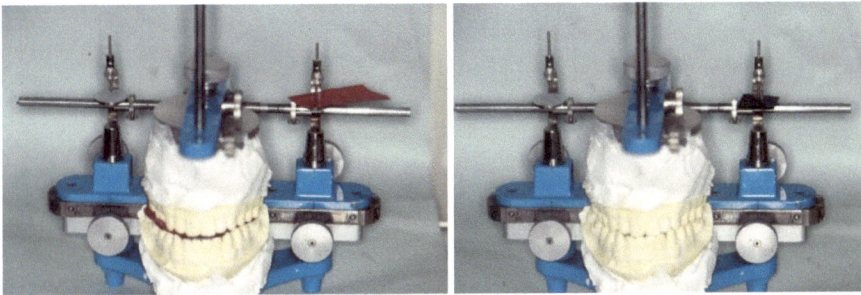

Figure 27: Occlusal analysis for the difference between HOP and BPOP.

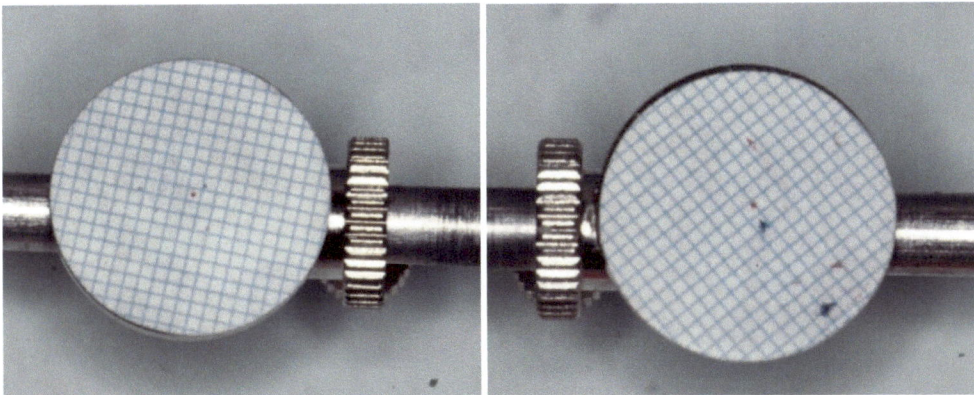

Figure 28: Recorded differences between HOP and BPOP.

The red points indicate the BPOP while the blue points indicate the HOP.

The premature contacts were examined on the articulator (Fig. **30**) and located on both molars of both sides (Fig. **31**). These premature contacts were removed on the casts and ground out in the patient's mouth while referring to their positions on the casts. Two weeks after removing the premature contacts in the BPOP, the patient still reported mild tenderness on palpation of the left sternocleidomastoideus and the external and medial pterygoideus muscles. Generally, complete disappearance of TMD signs and symptoms can be achieved with only occlusal equilibration of BPOP. However, because the patient still reported some muscle tenderness after occlusal adjustment of the BPOP, an occlusal analysis on lateral positions was performed (Figs. **32** and **33**).

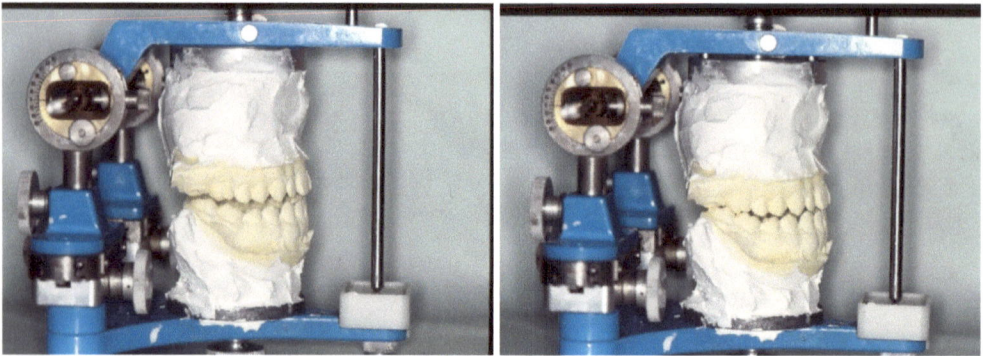

Figure 29: Reproduction of the MCP.

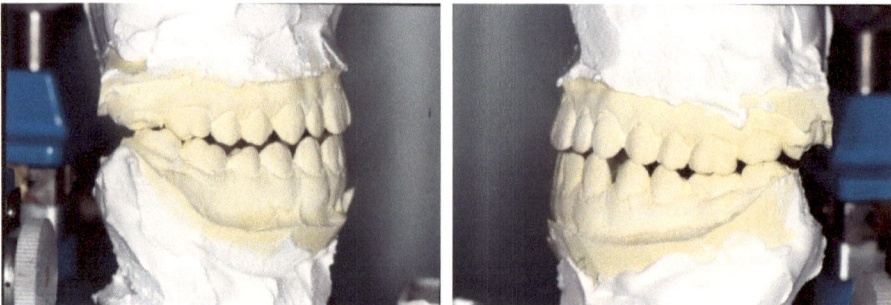

Figure 30: Lateral views of occlusion in the MCP.

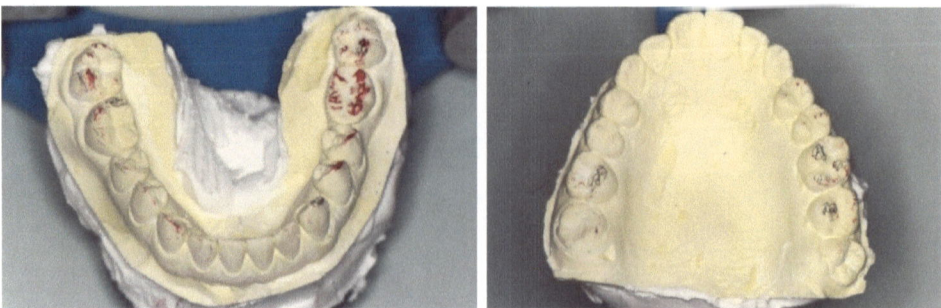

Figure 31: Removal of premature contacts.

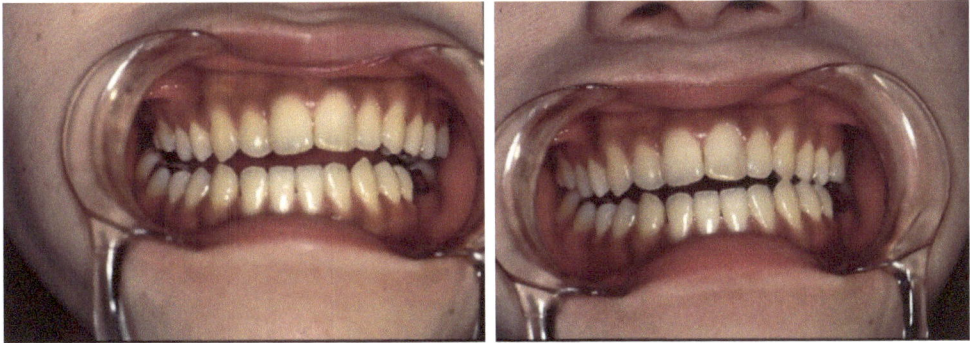

Figure 32: Occlusal relations in lateral positions.

The teeth on working side were unable to meet because of interferences on non-working side, particularly, on the right side (Fig. **32**).

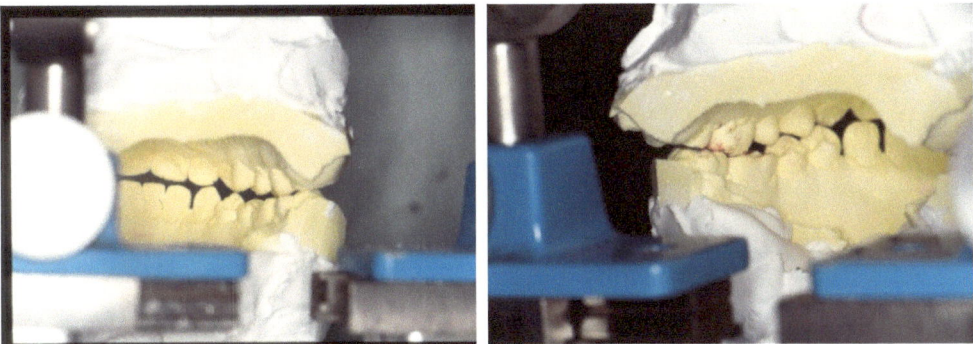

Figure 33: Interferences on non-working sides.

These interferences on non-working side were removed on the casts and ground in the patient's mouth (Fig. **34**).

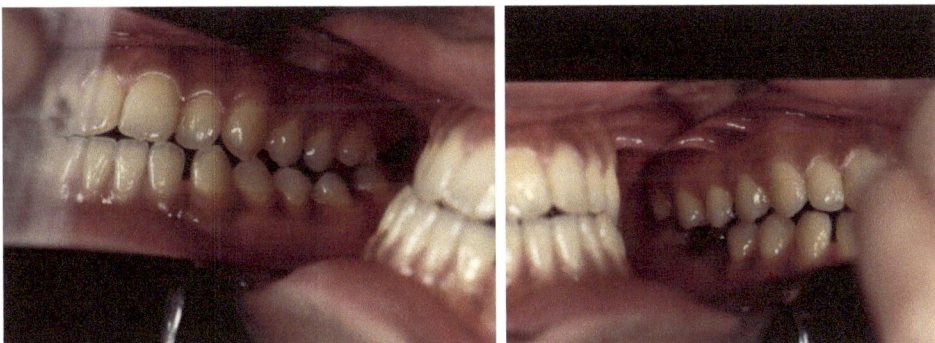

Figure 34: Lateral views of working sides.

After removing the interferences on the non-working sides, the muscle tenderness in the shoulder, neck and left occiput completely disappeared (Figs. **35** and **36**).

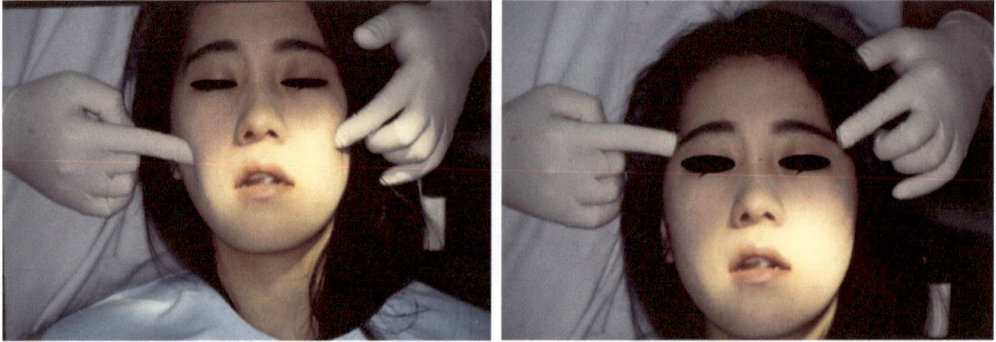

Figure 35: Complete disappearance of muscle tenderness.

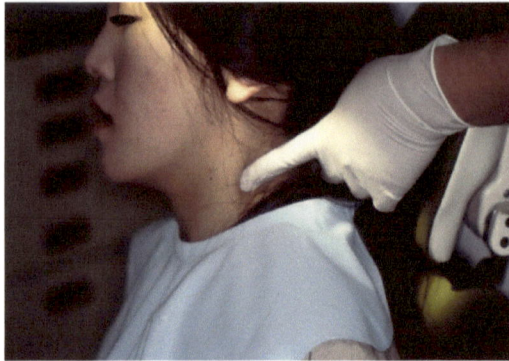

Figure 36: Palpation of sternocleidomastoideus.

The patient was completely recovered by 3 months of the first examination, and no recurrence of symptoms was observed over a 15-year follow-up period.

4. OCCLUSAL EQUILIBRATION USING PROSTHODONTIC OR ORTHODONTIC TREATMENT

Generally, two types of premature occlusal contacts occur in TMD patients: premature contact at the most posterior teeth with occlusion opening anteriorly (often seen in younger patients), and premature contact at the anterior teeth, with occlusion opening posteriorly (often seen in elderly patients). The former type should be treated only by occlusal adjustment, or sometimes using tooth

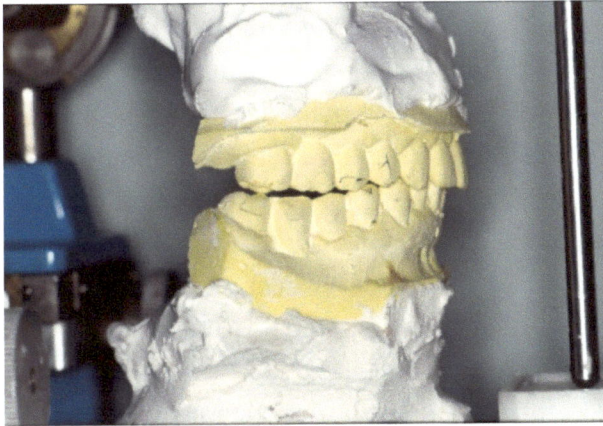

Figure 37: A wedge-shaped space in the right molar region.

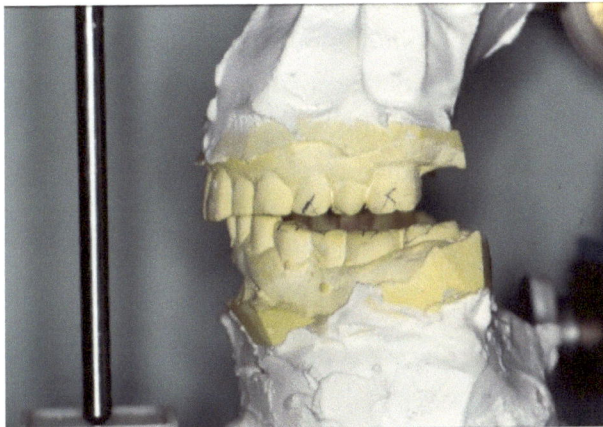

Figure 38: The wedge space was larger on the left than that on the right side.

reconstruction. However, for the latter type, it is necessary to build up an occlusion using full mouth reconstruction or orthodontic treatment. Rasmussen divided temporomandibular arthropathy into six phases on the basis of subjective symptoms. Phases 1 and 2 comprise of an initial stage of clicking and locking, phases 3 and 4 make up an intermediate stage of TMJ pain and constriction, and phases 5 and 6 make up the terminal stage. Phase 5 is characterized by non-painful residual symptoms and phase 6 by the complete disappearance of any subjective symptom (Rasmussen OC, 1981). In contrast, Nickerson and Boering stated that there is neither evidence that a joint with anteriorly displaced disk (ADR) with reduction must necessarily progress to the anteriorly displaced disk without reduction (ADNR), nor there is evidence that an arthritic reaction must develop in a joint with ADNR. In addition, an individual with an internal derangement and no pain may develop pain in future; however, the likelihood appears to diminish with age, particularly after 40 years of age. Those who attempt to apply remedial treatments directed toward internal derangements must take into consideration that almost all forms of therapy are approximately 80 % successful, and the same degree of success may result from "natural" events (Nickerson JW & Boering G, 1989). However, we have experienced many elderly patients with ADR without reduction. They were almost over 40 years of age (range, 38-76 years; mean, 56.1 ± 14.2 years), and they presented with major complaint of TMJ pain. The treatment periods ranged from 3 to 24 months, and the mean period was 9.0 ± 8.3 months. We now report a difficult case of TMJ disc displacement without reduction. A 50-year-old man presented with complaints of pain on the left TMJ and limited mouth opening. He underwent treatment comprising a combination of an occlusal splint and exposure of an infrared laser over 3 months, and after the symptoms resolved, a BPOP wax record was obtained and the casts were mounted on an articulator (Figs. **37** and **38**). Its was assumed that this occlusal relation may have occurred as a result of the stages 5 or 6 described by Ramussen (Rasmussen OC, 1981) (Fig. **39**).

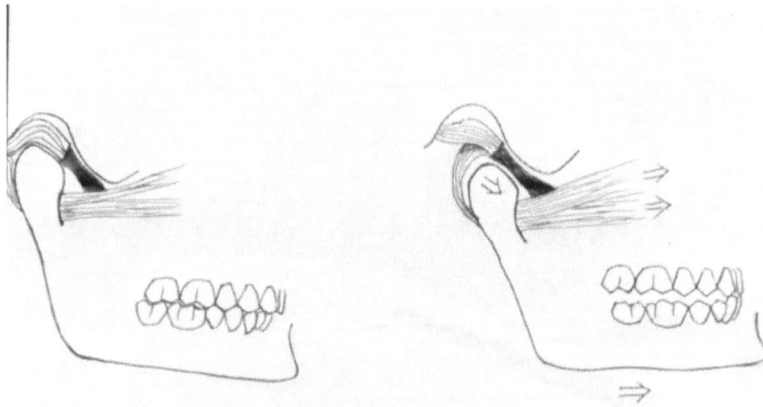

Figure 39: TMJ disc displacement without reduction on the right.

As the symptoms of TMD disappeared, the wedge shaped space appeared on the right.

The wedge shaped spaces on both sides had to be filled with something, and occlusion was induced with an occlusal flat plane splint to occlude all posterior teeth in this position without guidance from an anterior repositioning appliance. The wedge-shaped space was filled by occlusal reconstructions rather than by orthodontic therapy (Figs. **40** and **41**).

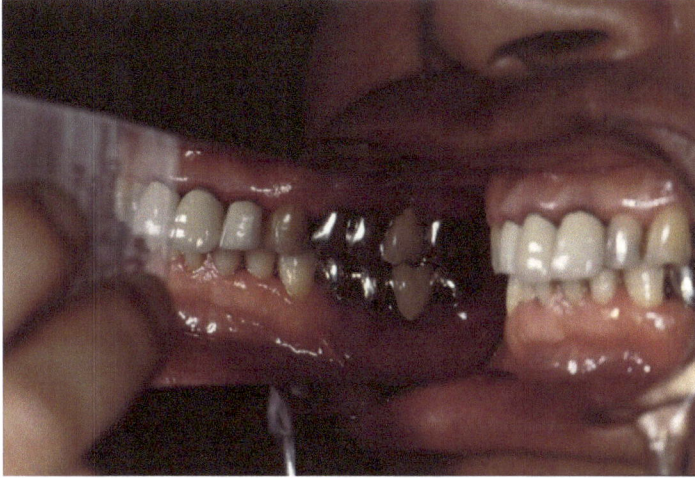

Figure 40: The wedge-shaped space on the right side. The space was filled with bridge works.

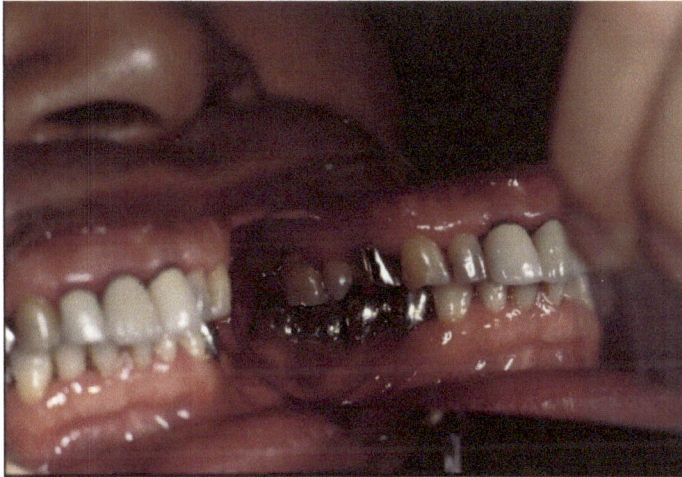

Figure 41: The wedge-shaped space on the left side. The space was filled with metal crowns.

Over a 16-year follow-up period, the lower prosthesis was replaced by a removable partial denture.

Brenkert described the orthodontic treatment to fill a wedge shaped space produced by anterior repositioning splint (Brenkert DR, 2010). He described the procedure in detail as follows. Orthodontic treatment for the anterior repositioned splint-stabilized patient following anterior disk displacement with resultant posterior openbite requires an organized and well-thought process. This technique uses the patient's current splint for continued stabilization because orthodontic treatment is undertaken. The next step is the need to have your orthodontic appliance having a lingual button on each posterior tooth (premolars/molars). The reason is the lingual cusps of the molars/premolars need positioning as the posterior teeth. Buccal elastics only do not adequately position the lingual cusps. The maxillary arch is then aligned while the patient continues to wear the mandibular splint. The splint is adjusted to allow tooth movement and the occlusal surface is realigned to maintain the anterior/posterior/medial/lateral position on every visit. This method eliminates the need to make a "Rickanator" type appliance and also the need to bond acrylic occlusal stops on the lower second molars. The Rickanator appliance has the drawbacks of food debris gathering under the acrylic, while the bite ramp size cannot be made large enough to maintain the stabilized A/P position, particularly at night. The occlusion on the Rickanator should be adjusted at each appointment; this necessitates its removal, resetting the occlusion, and reinsertion of the appliance. Bonding ramps on the lingual of the upper incisors are also eliminated, and the problem of adjusting the ramps as the mandibular anterior teeth are aligned is eliminated. Again, the lingual bonds cannot be made large enough to maintain the splinted position at night. Therefore, this technique uses a removable bite ramp that is worn at night only once the patient has the maxillary braces in place. The maxillary laterals are often undersized, and space orthodontically needs to be opened for the proper width of these teeth so that maxilla fits precisely over the mandible. All arch length discrepancies need to be resolved in the maxillary arch before initiating mandibular arch treatment. Once the maxillary teeth/arch is aligned, the next step is to reduce the splint from the mandibular second molars. Duration till the last step to align the second molars can prolong treatment and increase the risk of bite opening and recurrence of TMJ dysfunction. A light 3/16 inch, 4 1/2 oz. elastic is worn on buccal and lingual from the upper and lower second molars to align the lower second molar, considering that the upper second molar has already been aligned and that there is rectangular archwire to maintain the position of the upper second molar. Seating of the second molar is usually accomplished within 3-4 months. The splint maintains the vertical height and allows the alveolar bone in the region of the second molar to adapt to the new vertical height, without the molar having to assume a full occlusal load. The fourth step is to seat the mandibular anteriors (canine to canine). The splint is removed from the lower anteriors (canine to canine) and a sectional archwire is placed. These teeth are then aligned, and once a 16-round archwire is placed, 3/16 inch, 4 1/2 oz elastics are used to seat the anteriors and are worn 12-14 hours/day. The biteramp is adjusted to allow room for the mandibular anteriors to seat. This step usually takes 3-5 months. Once the anteriors are seated, a tripoded occlusal position is established and the daytime splint is discontinued. Step 5 involves the seating of premolars and first molars. The first molars and premolars are banded or bonded with brackets and lingual buttons. Elastics there to level the curve of Spee by erupting the first molars and premolars. Then, 5/16 inch, 4 oz. and/or 3/16 inch, 3 1/2 oz. elastics are used to seat the bite. A full lower archwire is placed once the first molars and premolars are touching occlusally, starting with a 16-round Nitinol archwire working up to a rectangular archwire. The biteramp is continued at night to protect from TMJ displacement and clenching and grinding. This stage averages 4-6 months. The final stage of treatment, step six, is details and finishes the occlusion. Anterior guidance is established with good lateral and protrusive movement. The importance of proper anterior guidance is critical to maintain the established condyle/disk position. Improper torque/positioning of the upper anterior teeth can result in an anterior incisal interference with recurrence of the original symptoms. This technique provides the practitioner with an easy straightforward method to wean a patient who has been on a splint for a displaced disk to a stabilized occlusal position, while maintaining the condyle/disk position established by the splint. The removable biteramp allows for greater flexibility. The ramp can be built large enough to maintain the A/P relationship needed at night. Patient cooperation and appreciation are enhanced because they can remove the biteramp during the day as they do not have to eat with it besides, they can brush and clean the appliance. The removable biteramp also allows for the treatment of Class III open bites. Sectionalizing the archwires allows for efficient tooth movement and light elastic forces to seat the bite. The average case can be successfully treated in 12-18 months. Retention is with removable wrap retainers with two Hawley maxillary wrap retainers and one

Hawley mandibular spring retainer. One maxillary retainer is constructed with a biteramp and is worn permanently at night, with the ramp adjusted so that the lower retainer can be worn ever at night with this retainer. The maxillary wrap retainer is worn during the day and discontinued after 6 months. It is important that the patient realizes the need to wear the retainers permanently at night (Brenkert DR, 2010). How long does it take to complete the orthodontic treatment, particularly in elderly patients with disc displacement without reduction? In filling the wedge-shaped space that appears when TMD symptoms are relieved, orthodontic treatment is advantageous because it is able to maintain the ratio of crown to root in each tooth. In prosthodontics treatment, the height of crown increases and the ratio becomes larger than the normal ratio. This condition is disadvantageous to support an occlusal load. The author does not agree with using an anterior repositioning appliance because disk displacement with reduction can be cured with occlusal equilibration in the MCP (BPOP). The wedge shaped-space appears in most cases of disk displacement without reduction once the symptoms disappeared.

SUMMARY

To obtain occlusal equilibration in the MCP, it is important to relieve the symptoms of TMDs prior to the equilibration and reproduce the MCP on dental casts mounted on an articulator and in the mouth. Before starting the occlusal adjustment, the premature contacts should be clearly explained to the patient, and the patient should also be shown the occlusal relation of the dental casts mounted on an articulator.

REFERENCES

Brenkert DR (2010). Orthodontic treatment for the TMJ patient following splint therapy to stabilize a displaced disk(s): A systemized approach. Part I, TMJ orthodontic diagnosis. *Cranio* 2010;28:193-199.

Brenkert DR (2010). Orthodontic treatment for the TMJ patient following splint therapy to stabilize a displacd disk(s): A systemized approach. Part II. *Cranio* 2010;28:260-265.

Dworkin SF, LeResch L (1992). Research diagnostic criteria for temporomandibular disorders. Review, criteria, examinations and specifications, critique. *J Craniomandib Disord Facial Oral Pain* 1992;6:310-355.

Nickerson JW & Boering G (1989). Natural course of osteoarthrosis as it relates to internal derangement of the temporomandibular joint. *Oral Maxillofac Surg Clin North Am* 1989;127-45.

Rasmussen OC (1981). Clinical findings during the course of temporomandibular arthropathy. *Scand J Dent Res* 1989;89:283-288.

Torii K (1989). Analysis of rotation centers of various mandibular closures. *J Prosthet Dent* 1989;61:285-291.

Torii K & Chiwata I (2010). Occlusal adjustment using the bite plate-induced occlusal position as a reference position for temporomandibular disorders: a pilot study. *Head & Face Medicine* 2010;6:5. Available from: http://www.head-face-med.com/content/6/1/5

Send Orders for Reprints to reprints@benthamscience.net

CHAPTER 8

Possible Mechanism of Temporomandibular Disorders

Abstract: Regarding the mechanism of temporomandibular disorders (TMDs), TMD pain including muscle tenderness to palpation is considered to be caused by masticatory muscle fatigue induced with occlusal discrepancy. Temporomandibualr joint (TMJ) derangement is considered to be occurred due to mandibular displacement from muscular position to habitual position.

Keywords: TMJ derangement, muscle fatigue, muscle tenderness, muscle spasm, masticatory muscles, neuralgias, earache, jawache, ethyl chloride spray, tensional factors, malocclusion, disc displacement, myofascial pain, capsulitis, trigger point, postural habits, vascular headache, nociceptor, occlusal discrepancy.

1. INTRODUCTION

Since Schwartz described that TMDs are supposed to be caused with muscle spasm, many studies on masticatory muscles and other involved muscles have been performed. Schwartz described as follows:

Two hundred and fifty-six patients, mainly women, suffering from symptoms associated with the temporomandibular joint, were examined at the Temporomadibular Joint Clinic, a research clinic of the School of Dental and Oral Surgery, at the Columbia-Presbyterian Medical Center. The symptom-complex described by Costen was not found. Pain and dysfunction in the form of limitation of mandibular movement were the symptoms most frequently encountered in this group of patients, reported in 1954. The pain described by these patients differed from the sudden, paroxysmal and irregular pain of the neuralgias. It was usually described as a unilateral, constant, dull earache or jawache initiated or aggravated by jaw movements and sometimes spreading to the head, neck, and shoulder. Diagnostic surveys, with the cooperation of many departments of the Medical Center, disclosed extremely low incidence of temporomandibular joint disease (less than 3 per cent). Muscle tenderness was often found among patients suffering from temporomandibular joint pain and dysfunction. This tenderness was located in various antigravity muscles of the jaws, neck, and shoulder (masseter, internal pterygoid, temporalis, posterior cervical, and trapezius) as well

Kengo Torii

as the sternomastoid. The nature of the symptoms, dull ache with limitation of movement, suggested a pain-spasm cycle of the type described by Travell and Kraus. The effectiveness of ethyl chloride spray and of intramuscular infiltration with a local anesthetic followed by the exercising of the masticatory muscles supported this conclusion. Continuing studies are confirming the 1954 findings. In a recent amplified four-year study, 377 (77.8 per cent) of 491 patients examined (398 female and 93 male) presented symptoms in the form of a complex-a temporomandibular joint pain-dysfunction syndrome. This syndrome often was precipitated by sudden or continuous stretch of the masticatory muscles, as in a yawn, wide bite, dental treatment, or by proprioceptive changes caused by sudden or extensive alterations in the dental occlusion through treatment. Predisposition, psychologic as well as physiologic, seem to be more important than the particular form of the precipitating factor itself. Tensional factors were evident among many patients, some of whom had psychiatric interviews. Emotional tension was often manifested by a history of oral habits such as clenching or gnashing the teeth. Dental malocclusion in the group studied was too universal and varied to permit detailed evaluation. It is believed however, that malocclusion in most cases was but a contributing factor (Schwartz LL, 1956). On the other hand, the studies on TMJ disc displacement (internal derangement) are not sufficient regarding the etiology. The mechanism of muscle pain or myofascial pain has been cleared to some extent, however, the causes or factors of TMJ disc displacement remain unclear.

2. POSSIBLE MECHANISM OF MYOFASCIAL PAIN

Fricton *et al.* reviewed the clinical characteristics of 164 patients whose chief complaints led to the diagnosis of myofascial pain syndrome (MPS), and reported that these patients had (1) tenderness at points in firm bands of skeletal muscle that were consistent with past reports, (2) specific pattern of pain referral associated with each trigger point, (3) frequent emotional, postural, and behavioral contributing factors, and (4) frequent associated symptoms and concomitant diagnoses (Fricton JR, 1985). They described as follows: Myofascial pain syndrome was the primary diagnosis in 164 of 296 patients (55.4%) and accounted for the highest percentage of any diagnosis. The other primary diagnosis found included TMJ internal derangement with capsulitis (41, 13.9%),

TMJ degenerative joint disease with capsulitis (21, 7.1%), vascular headaches (19, 6.4%), continuous or paroxysmal trigeminal neuralgia (14, 4.7%), and other diagnoses (37, 12.4%). Trigger points with associated referral patterns of pain were found in most muscles of the head and neck and ranged between 2 mm and 5 mm in diameter. The patterns of pain referral were consistent with patterns of other patients with similar trigger points. Acute cases of MPS generally displayed pain only at the trigger point, but as the disease became more chronic it increased to distant and multiple areas. This study supports a multifactorial etiologic basis for MPS. Patients reported the onset of pain to be related to both macrotraumatic and microtraumatic events. Macrotrauma, such as physical trauma to the muscle due to acute strain or direct injury, was found in minority of cases to be the initiating event. Microtraumatic behaviors, such as sustained contraction during oral parafunctional habits, muscle tension, and poor postural habits, may have played a role in the gradual development of trigger points. Poor postural habits, such as maintenance of a forward head position, require muscles to sustain contraction to counteract forces of gravity. Once trigger points develop, the muscle becomes restricted and painful when stretched; this causes the patient to protect the muscle through continued poor posturing and sustained contraction. This may perpetuate the trigger point and develop other trigger points in the same muscle and in agonist muscles. Factors that have been suggested to weaken the muscle and predispose it to the development of trigger points were common. This included poor structural imbalances, such as occlusal disharmonies, lack of adequate sleep, and the presence of other disorders. Occlusal disharmonies may cause condylar displacement and occlusal avoidance patterns, resulting in abnormal proprioceptive input and sustained muscle contraction in attempt to correct the poor postural relationships of the jaws and allow harmonious function. Other disorders found in association with MPS, such as TMJ internal derangement, vascular headaches, and neuralgias, may cause nociceptive input to the central nervous system that stimulates motor unit activity in the area of the pain, setting up a reverberatory circuit that may lead to the development of trigger points in the muscles. Forty-two of these patients also reported sleep problems, supporting the theory that MPS may be a sleep disturbance syndrome that predisposes the patient to the development of trigger point. Although the pathophysiology of MPD is yet to be confirmed, the concepts presented here with theories proposed by Simons and Travell, Melzack, and Awad may help stimulate further understanding of this phenomenon. Etiologic factors, including macrotraumatic or microtraumatic events, may strain the muscles through muscle injury (whiplash, excess jaw opening, *etc.*). These traumas release free calcium within the muscle through disruption of the sarcoplasmic reticulum and, with ATP, stimulate actin and myosin interaction and local contractile and metabolic activity. This activity, if continued, may lead to release of substances, such as serotonin, histamine, kinins, and prostaglandins, that sensitize and fire Groups III and IV muscle nociceptors and pain perception results. If this pain results in further muscle contraction through posturing or habits, a reverberatory neural circuit is established between the nociceptors, the central nervous system, and the motor units. These afferent nociceptive inputs may converge with other visceral and somatic inputs in the cells, such as those of the lamina V of the dorsal horn or the substantia gelatinosa on the way to the cortex, and result in the perception of referred pain. These inputs may be facilitated or inhibited by peripheral or central influences at the "central biasing mechanism" of the brainstem. Various treatment modalities, such as cold, heat analgesic medications, massage, trigger point injections, and transcutaneous electrical stimulation, may diminish the reverberatory cycle and reduce pain. Likewise, the cycle may be perpetuated by continued protective splinting of the painful muscle through both distorted muscle posture and avoidance of painful stretching of the muscles or by further sustained neural activity through continued parafunctional habits or inputs from pathologic viscera or dysfunctional joints. With contractile activity sustained, local blood flow is decreased, resulting in depleted ATP reserves and diminished calcium pump. Free calcium continues to interact with ATP to trigger contractile activity, especially if actin and myosin are overlapping within the shortened muscle, and a self-perpetuating cycle is established. Sustained increases in the local noxious substances then contribute to inflammation within the interstitial connective tissue at the trigger point and further disrupt III of the calcium pump. If normal muscle length is not restored through exercise and improved posture and the pain continues, behavioral and psychosocial disturbances may further perpetuate the problem. If the process continues, the muscle band initially attempts to respond with hypertrophy but later breaks down to granular ground substance, eventually resulting in localized fibrosis (Fricton JR, 1985). Stohler described as follows: No single model of the causation of muscle-related TMD has emerged to be the most valid at this time. *Peripheral sensitization.* There is a lowered response threshold of nociceptors to mechanical and thermal stimuli in the state of inflammation or tissue damage. This so-called peripheral sensitization of nociceptive afferents is in contrast to the adaptive changes that occur in other somatosensory systems with continued stimulus presentation. The altered response characteristic is attributed to a range of chemical mediators that are released from damaged tissue cells, mast cells, platelets, or the nociceptors themselves, and can either activate (eg, histamine, bradykinin, serotonin, potassium) or sensitize (eg, substance P, prostaglandins, leukotrienes) free nerve endings. Nociceptors can also be activated by sympathetic stimulation following sensitization by an injury or inflammation. Increasing the complexity of possible interactions, newer data suggest that endogenous opioid peptides are synthesized by inflammatory cells, which may be a mechanism by which anti-nociception is exerted in peripheral tissues. In the context of peripheral sensitization, increasing interest focuses on nerve growth factor (NFG) as a mediator in persistent muscle pain. Besides the role of NGF as a target-derived trophic factor in early ontogeny, it was shown that small adult primary sensory neurons, particularly those that contain calcitonin gene-related peptide, express the high-affinity NGF receptor trkA. Systemic application of NGF causes hyperalgesia in both neonatal and adult rats. Pretreatment with NGF antibody reduces or prevents carrageenan-induced arthritis in rats. Because healthy volunteers developed pain in the bulbar, jaw, and truncal musculature following intravenous injection of NGF, this secretory protein appears to be important in the pathogenesis of muscle related TMD. Human volunteers injected with NGF described the experience as "muscle overuse pain", and women seemed to experience pain for a longer time than men. Indeed, estrogen has been shown to up-regulate trkA messenger RNA, thereby affecting the efficiency of NGF binding. This could be one of the reasons for the increased persistence and severity of muscle pain conditions among women. Nerve growth factor has also been shown to stimulate the production of substance P, somatostatin, and vasoactive intestinal polypeptide in sensory neurons and affects inflammatory cells that express the trkA receptor, such as mast cells. As mast cells are known to exist in the perimysium of muscle, and mast cell degranulation has been shown to occur in muscle soreness following strenuous muscle work, there is a real possibility that NGF-related peripheral effects contribute to clinical muscle pain conditions. *Central neuroplasticity and sensitization.* A great benefit can be gained from conceptualizing the clinical muscle pain conditions in the context of neuroplasticity and central sensitization. Regarding neuroplasticity, a distinction is made between neural and behavioral plasticity. Neuroplasticity refers to the reorganization of the nervous system based on mechanisms that influence synaptic efficacy and connectivity at all levels of the brain. Both short-term (lasting minutes) and long-term (lasting for hours and longer) changes are distinguished. Examples of behavioral plasticity include sensitization, habituation, and rehabilitation. Sensitization describes the phenomenon of an enhanced behavioral response; habituation, on the other hand, refers to the decrease in the behavioral response with repeated stimulus applications. At the level of cellular networks, a decrease in the synaptic strength forms the basis of habituation, whereas sensitization involves the greater availability of excitatory neurotransmitter in the synaptic cleft. Neuroplasticity and sensitization provide the basis for maching the response to the local condition in terms of injury detection, pain avoidance, pain escape, and the need for rest of the injured body part to promote recuperation. Although neuroplasticity and sensitization have a purpose in the context of survival function, the very same mechanisms seem to be involved in the generation of symptoms and signs that dominate the clinical picture of muscle-related TMD. With their first synapse, nociceptive afferents arising from the jaw and neck musculature connect to projection neurons and inhibitory or excitatory interneurons. The significant convergence of afferent input at this level explains the spread and referral of pain. In addition to nociceptive input, non-nociceptive afferents and descending anti-nociceptive systems may influence the exitability of these neurons as well. Different neurotransmitters (*e.g.* glutamate, aspartate, and substance P) are implicated in evoking both fast and slow synaptic potentials by acting on NMDA, AMPA (glutamic acid receptors), and neurokinin-1 receptors. Among the excitatory neurotransmitters, substance P, an 11-amino-acid neuropeptide, has been receiving most attention because of its perceived relevance in conditions of persistent muscle pain. Studies in humans have shown that substance P levels in the cerebrospinal fluid are elevated in FMS patients when compared with controls. Allodynia which is a key feature of muscle -related TMD, is associated with increased exitability of rat dorsal horn neurons during spinal cord superfusion with substance P. The increased exitability that is paralleled by enlargement of mechanoreceptive fields of the second-order neurons is an expression of the inflammation-induced neuroplasticity. *Pro-Nociceptive pathways.* Nociceptive information arising from the muscles of the head and neck is relayed *via* the spinal cord and corresponding structures of the trigeminal brain stem complex to subcortical and cortical centers. A direct pathway, which connects with nuclei in the lateral part of the thalamus, is primarily made up of ascending input from spinal or trigeminal laminae I and V. Deeper layers (laminae VI, VII, and VIII) contribute to an indirect pain pathway, which targets the reticular formation before establishing a connection with nuclei in the medial portion of the thalamus. The latter system is implicated in influencing hormone release from the hypothalamus and pituitary gland and is known to affect supraspinal autonomic reflexes. It is quite clear that the neurosecretory function of a particular cell type is not regulated by a single neurotransmitter. Instead, the response of hypothalamic neurosecretory cells is dependent on a combination of neurotransmitters, with hormones acting as modulators. Evidence further suggests that the lateral or direct pathway carries predominantly the sensory-discriminative information of pain, while the indirect or medial pain pathway is associated with more affective-motivational aspects of pain. At the cortical level, the primary somatosensory cortex is the target of the sensory discriminative information content of pain, and there is evidence that the frontal lobe is linked to pain and unpleasantness. All this is relevant because certain therapies have been shown to exert differential effects in these 2 systems. *Anti-Nociceptive pathway.* Descending inhibitory influences are exerted from the cortex, diencephalon, areas such as the periaqueductal gray and periventricular gray in the midbrain, and the medulla on nociceptive neurons in the subnucleus caudalis or spinal dorsal horn. Nociceptive neurons with input predominantly from deep tissues appear to be especially influenced by such descending control, with the evidence further suggesting that the anti-nociceptive influences are greater in tonic pain than in acute pain. Endogenous opioid peptides and serotonin are implicated in mediating these inhibitory, anti-nociceptive effects. High levels of substance P in the spinal cord are associated with low brain serotonin levels in rats. In humans, low concentrations of endogenous opioids in the cerebrospinal fluid have been reported in persistent painful neuropathy. Antidepressants that demonstrate an analgesic effect when compared with placebo are believed to exert this influence by facilitating pain-inhibiting pathways. *Neuroendocrine and autonomic stress response.* Because abnormality in neuroendocrine function exists in depressed persons, it has been suggested that stress-induced dysfunction of the HPA (hypothalamic-pituitary-adrenal) system is a factor in FMS (fibromyalgia syndrome) and possibly other related pain condition in which depressive symptoms are prevalent. As far as the stress is concerned, two major response patterns are distinguished. The acute response supports the defense reaction; the chronic response pattern elicits a vigilance reaction. Complex neuroendocrine and autonomic mechanisms are in effect to influence any stress-induced deviation from homeostasis, with the hypothalamus forming the major link between the CNS, the HPA axis, and the supraspinal autonomic reflex centers. Environmental stimuli and emotional and cognitive factors influence the hypothalamic neurosecretory cells that regulate the release of neurohormones (*e.g.* corticotropin-releasing hormone), which in turn affect the synthesis of hormones by the pituitary gland. Synthesis of peripheral hormones, such as cortisol from the adrenal cortex, is under pituitary control by way of adrenocorticotropin. To increase complexity, hypothalamic and pituitary neurohormones have not only peripheral but also central targets, which include altering the expression of neurotransmitter receptors and, thereby affecting the neural regulation of autonomic reflexes, behavior, and emotional states. For example, corticotropin-releasing hormone is implicated in increasing arousal and emotionality, and adrenocorticotropin facilitates attention. On the other hand, inputs from the cerebrospinal fluid and circulatory system (hormone, neuropeptides, *etc.*) function as feedback signals that affect the release of neurotransmitters and adjust the hypothalamic release of neurohormones. In view of stress being a poorly defined construct and the highly interactive nature of the neuroendocrine system, cause-and-effect questions are difficult to resolve in clinical cases of muscle pain. Insight into the role of the HPA axis is further complicated by the fact that cortisol is secreted in a circadian rhythm, with the lowest levels occurring at midnight and the highest levels at about 8 in the morning, calling for hourly sampling to track levels in serum. As the newer findings also suggest that the nature of the HPA response system is specific for a particular type of stressor, greater care is applicable in the synthesis of the literature. If the current stress construct, which is based on the assumption of non-specificity in the response to wide range of stressors, is no longer valid, many generalizations about catecholaminergic activation will no longer appropriate. Although neuroendocrine functions appear to be highly relevant in muscle-related TMD, detailed studies of the nature of their contribution to the pathogenesis of symptoms and signs in the TMD are not yet available (Stohler CS, 1999).

Torii and Chiwata reported the outcome of occlusal adjustment using the bite plate-induced occlusal position as a reference position based on the evidence that there was a significant relation between the occlusal discrepancy (discrepancy between HOP and BPOP) and TMJ sounds (Torii K & Chiwata I, 2010). However, the cause-and-effect relation between the occlusal discrepancy and TMDs has not been demonstrated, because it is difficult to create an artificial occlusal discrepancy in human subject as the occlusal discrepancy might emerge in a long period as shown in Torri's longitudinal study (Torii K, 2011). In Torii's study, the incidence of TMJ clicking was mostly temporarily, but a few subjects had persistent clicking after the intermittent incidence. At the stage of this persistent clicking, it was supposed that the occlusal discrepancy had been established. Therefore, it is supposed that creating an artificial occlusal discrepancy is very difficult in human subject. Since the occlusal adjustment with eliminating the occlusal discrepancy was effective for myofascial pain as well as for TMJ disc displacement, it is supposed that the occlusal discrepancy between the habitual occlusal position (HOP) and the bite plate-induce occlusal position (BPOP) might be related to the cause of myofascial pain (Torii K& Chiwata I, 2010). The cause-and- effect relation between the occlusal discrepancy and TMDs is thought to be indirectly demonstrated. The existence of an occlusal discrepancy between the HOP and BPOP means that when the mandible voluntarily closes, the elevator muscles require additional activity to adapt the mandible from the BPOP to the HOP as multiple teeth come in contact with stable position during isotonic muscle contraction to isometric. This condition may cause muscle fatigue, resulting in muscle pain. The elimination of such a discrepancy through occlusal adjustment reduces the activity of the muscles and consequently reduces and alleviates the painful symptoms of TMDs, as reported in the study by Torii and Chiwata (Torii K& Chiwata I, 2010). Regarding fatigue in human jaw muscle, Mao *et al.* described as follows: *Central fatigue* involves a failure of the command associated with the motor cortex and the upper motoneuron. The central nervous system reduces its motor drive (*e.g.* the subject is "tired of continuing"), but the peripheral elements of the nerve and the muscle fibers are unimpaired. More force could be generated by voluntary effort or by directly stimulating the muscle. *Peripheral fatigue* affects components of the command chain distal to and including the motor end plate. It may be caused by a disruption in either transmission or contraction. *Transmission fatigue* is caused by a failure either at the motor end plate or in the postsynaptic propagation of the electrical impulse along the cell membrane, including its extensions into the T-tubules, of a muscle fiber. *Contraction fatigue* is due to either a failure to convert the extracellular electrical transmission into an intracellular chemical reaction or to a failed link in the chain of these intracellular reactions, the end result of which is to cause the actin and myosin filaments to slide across each other. Fatigue can be induced either by sustained voluntary contractions or by electrically stimulating a motor nerve or the muscle itself. Electrical stimulation can produce two types of fatigue, depending on the frequency at which the nerve or muscle is stimulated. *Low-frequency fatigue* corresponds to contraction fatigue and is the result of stimulation below approximately 20 Hz (20 stimuli per second). It takes a long time to develop and the recovery is slow. *High-frequency fatigue* corresponds to transmission fatigue and is the result of stimulation above approximately 80 Hz. It is quickly induced and the recovery is rapid. Studies of jaw muscle fatigue have, as yet, been limited. All members of a synergistic group of muscles should be simultaneously monitored because a reduced activity in one may be compensated by an increased activity in another. If only the occlusal force is being measured (and sustained) then, prior to the failure point, other signs are hidden and the only indication of progressive fatigue is discomfort or pain. Medial pterygoid activity has rarely been studied because it is only accessible to needle electrodes. Furthermore, all the jaw closing muscles contain differently oriented elements that can operate independently. The deep elements are also inaccessible to surface EMG measurements. Occlusal forces have only been monitored with unidirectional force transducers, which measure the component of the force parallel to a measuring axis. Using a three-dimensional occlusal force transducer Osborn and Mao have shown that the early anterior direction of an incisal occlusal force changes to nearly vertical at the end of the maximum voluntary contraction. An apparent change in the magnitude of the occlusal force measured by a unidirectional transducer may in reality be partially due to a change in its direction. This may also account for some discrepancies between the results of previous studies. Human jaw muscles contain different propotions of fast and slow fibers. Henneman's size principle states that when a muscle contracts with increasing force, slow motor units are recruited first, followed by fast motor units. This orderly recruitment pattern has been shown to exist in jaw muscles. The fast fibers in jaw muscles are usually recruited for stronger forces. Histochemical studies have consistently suggested that human jaw closing muscles contain rather more fatigue-resistant slow fibers (type I) than fatigue-susceptible fast fibers (type IIB). The electrical responses to fatigue of these two types of fiber in jaw muscles, however, have only been tested once. In limb muscles type I and type II fibers have been shown to have different glycogen depletion patterns and this suggests that the rate at which they lose force (*i.e.* their fatigability) is also different. Histochemical studies also indicated that there are very few fast-contracting, fatigue-resistant (type II A) fibers in human jaw closing muscles. These are abundant in ruminants such as cattle and sheep, animals that spend much of their waking life chewing. The near absence of type IIA fibers from human jaw muscles seems to suggest that they would be readily susceptible to fatigue during sustained effort at stronger force levels because fast, fatigue-susceptible (type IIB) fibers must be recruited at these levels. Mao *et al.* suggested that the existing proportions of fiber types in human jaw muscles may be recent and associated with the change to an increasingly softer and less challenging diet. It could have been important for earlier human populations to be able to maintain prolonged jaw activity while breaking up tough low-energy food or while chewing on leather to soften it. Part of the change would have been a decrease in the number of fast, fatigue-resistant, type IIA fibers. The pain described by Clark and coworkers could be a protective mechanism, related to this decrease, which prematurely affects some temporomandibular disorder subjects (Mao J *et al.*, 1993). On the other hand, Glaros *et al.* examined the role of parafunctional clenching on various measures of TMD pain (Glaros AG *et al.*, 1998). In their study, five subjects participated in daily 17-minute electromyogram biofeedback training sessions structured in three phases. Subjects were instructed to maintain temporalis and masseter muscle activity below 2 µV in the first (decrease) phase of training (10 sessions), above 10 µV in the second (increase) phase (1 to 8 sessions), and below

$2\mu V$ in the third (decrease) phase (10 to 15 sessions). Preliminary screening examinations showed that none of the subject had TMD. Two subjects reported intolerable pain during increase training, and both were diagnosed with TMD pain during this phase. No subject was diagnosed with TMD pain during either decrease training phase. They are described as follows: Two of the five subjects, both women, terminated increase training early because of self-reported intolerable pain. These findings suggest that the experimental protocol succeeded in increasing TMD pain in a subset of the subjects who participated in this study. A variety of factors might account for the presence of pain in this subset of subjects, including differing levels of pain tolerance, differing levels of muscle activity during increase trials, and differing biochemical/physiologic responses in the musculature to sustained, low-level activity. All three of the women participated in this study used oral contraceptives, and the use of these medications may have increased their susceptibility to experimental clenching. Considerably, more research would be needed to identify the characteristics of individuals who responded with pain to the protocol used here. The possibility that experimenter bias and subject expectation effects were in part responsible for the results on pain should also be considered. The findings from this study suggest that low-level parafunctional activity may be a mechanism of producing pain in some TMD patients. According to this model, some were engaged in low-level parafunctional activity for lengthy periods of time. The activity might consist of tooth contact, more intense clenching, or other kinds of parafunction. In any case, the activity of the masseter and other elevator muscles is likely to be significantly greater than the activity recorded when the muscles are at rest. The data from the present study suggest that this low-level activity can result in arthralgia or a myofascial pain. The 17 minites of daily training performed by these subjects (for a maximum of 8 days) may be only a minor approximation of the amount of time that some TMD patients engage in parafunctional activities. Unfortunately, nonreactive, *in vivo* measures of parafunctional clenching in TMD patients are not available. Individuals diagnosed with myofascial pain appear to have deficits in proprioceptive awareness, and this may account for their failure to recognize that they engage in parafunctional activity. In further research, it would be useful to identify the factors that distinguish individuals who respond with pain to the experimental protocol from those who do not (Glaros AG *et al.*, 1998). It is supposed that this increase phase produced muscle fatigue itself. Unconsciously continued effort to adapt the mandible to the HOP from the BPOP may cause myofascial pain. Svensson and Graven-Nielsen described as follows: in conditions with heavy loading and insufficient relaxation period, concentric dynamic and isometric contractions will produce muscle pain that probably involves the same pathologic process as ischemic pain. Ischemia alone is not sufficient to evoke muscle pain, but in combination with contractions, strong pain develops in humans. Accumulation of metabolites such as lactate, potassium, or the lack of oxidation of metabolic products, in addition to mechanical factors (*e.g.*, the number of contractions, their duration and force), may play a significant role. A combination of concentric dynamic contractions, *e.g.*, mastication and ischemic block of the superficial temporal artery, produces a continuously increasing dull, bilateral, frontal headache in healthy subjects. Sustained or repeated static tooth-clenching tasks in different jaw positions may also lead to intense jaw muscle pain with a rapid onset. It is notable that pain disappears quickly when clenching ceases, and most studies in healthy subjects have failed to show clinically significant levels of pain in the jaw muscles in the days following exercise. In contrast to the immediate and rather short-lasting muscle pain evoked by concentric contraction, eccentric contractions are more effective in inducing a delayed onset of muscle pain or soreness in limb muscles. The mechanism underlying this kind of muscle pain is probably related to damage to muscle connective tissue. Thus, the result of exercise-induced activation of human muscle nociceptors shows that excessive and strong contractions of the muscles can cause pain in the craniofacial region, but the pain is usually short-lasting and self-limiting. Furthermore, due to the nature of the experimental procedures, there may be a strong confounding factor of muscle fatigue. In addition, muscle pain is usually developed in a group of muscle synergists rather than in one specific muscle. Other techniques are therefore required to allow the study of both somatosensory effects of pain and the sensorimotor integration in the craniofacial region, and they are summarized as follows: The factor that causes craniofacial muscle pain in the first place is still unknown, but it seems clear that there is no single or simple cause in the majority of cases. There is no indication of a genetic predisposition for the development of TMD pain. Thus, in current multifactorial models of TMD pain, a series of initiating, predisposing, and aggravating biochemical, neuromuscular biopsychosocial, and neurobiologic factors has been considered. A recent hypothesis has highlighted some of the neurobiologic factors, such as an interaction between NGF and estrogen levels. If jaw muscles are injured by accident or during function, this could trigger a sequence of critical events in the peripheral tissue that lead to sensitization of afferent channels and perhaps even cause reorganization at the cortical level. Further studies are needed to identify the factors responsible for the initiation of the events and for the transition from acute to persistent muscle pain. The experimental pain studies presented in this review have at this point contributed to a more advanced understanding of both the somatosensory and motor effects of craniofacial muscle pain and added further causion to strict biomechanical thinking with untimely overemphasis on, for example, dental occlusion. Tonic experimental jaw muscle pain has been shown to directly change the occlusal relationship, which challenges the etiologic importance of occlusal factors in the development of TMD pain. Thus, it seems appropriate that treatment should be guided towards the management of pain rather than restoration of motor "dysfunction". Moreover, pain management should be directed both to the peripheral tissue, where pain may be initiated, and to the central nervous system, where pain is maintained. A pharmacologic approach using molecules with dual drug actions may be one way amongst others in future to pursue the goal of effective pain management. It is evident that human experimental pain research alone cannot solve the puzzle of persistent muscle pain in the craniofacial region, but it can be used to test and generate specific questions, which is not possible in animal or clinical research. Thus, human experimental pain research should remain a bridge between basic animal research and cotrolled clinical trials (Svensson P & Graven-Nielsen T, 2001). In their summary, they referred to the article of McNamara *et al.* (it has been also referred in Chapter 3) (McNamara JA *et al.*, 1995), and in the summary of the article, they described as follows: Signs and symptoms of TMD occur in healthy individuals and increase with age, particularly during adolescents; thus TM disorders that originate during various types of dental treatment may not be related to the treatment but may be a naturally occurring phenomenon. The author partly demonstrated their description: Persistent TMJ clicking occurred at an age of 11 or 12 years in not related to dental treatment (see Chapter 1) (Torii K, 2011). In addition, Svensson and Graven-Nielsen referred to the article of Obrez and Stohler (Obrez A & Stohler CS, 1996), and in their study they provided evidence of an alternative causal relationship between pain and changes in occlusal relationship.

In contrast with this, Torii and Chiwata demonstrated the relation between occlusal discrepancy and TMD sign (TMJ clicking) without any pain (Torii K & Chiwata I, 2005). In addition, Torii and Chiwata reported that the relation between occlusal discrepancy and TMD symptoms existed without pain (see Chapter 4) (Torii K & Chiwata I, 2010). The bite force in a mastication seems to be smaller than those in these experimental clenching (as described in the review of Svensson & Graven-Nielsen), but the accumulative muscle fatigue due to the additional activity to adapt the mandible to the HOP from the BPOP may cause muscle pain. On the other hand, Dao and Lavigne investigated pain responses to experimental chewing in myofascial pain patients. In their study, pain was assessed before and after chewing wax for 3 minutes, in 20 asymptomatic subjects (control) and in 61 patients with muscle pain. They reported as follows: No asymptomatic subjects had pain before and after the chewing test, while about 50% of the patients reported an increase in pain after chewing. In this subgroup, mean pain intensity increased by 102.6%. However, mean pain intensity after chewing decreased by 56.6% in about 30% of the patients. These patients had significantly higher resting pain than the first subgroup. These data show that even a short chewing test can exacerbate pain in most myofascial pain patients but it has no effect on asymptomatic subjects. Surprisingly, the exercise decreases pain in an important subgroup of patients. These results suggest that two subgroups of myofascial pain patients may exist with opposite reactions to exercise. It remains to be observed if these reactions are due to two different pathologies or to the fact that the pre-exercise pain levels were significantly different in the two groups (Dao TTT *et al.*, 1994).

3. POSSIBLE MECHANISM OF TMJ DISC DISPLACEMENT

In the study of occlusal adjustment of Tori and Chiwata, TMJ clicking disappeared by making the HOP consistent with the BPOP by eliminating the premature occlusal contacts in the BPOP (Torii K& Chiwata I, 2010). From this fact, it is supposed that the correct relation between the TMJ disc and the condyle is distorted with the premature contacts in TMD patient. When the mandible closes, the condyle is moved backward by the sliding movement of the mandible from the muscular postion to a more stable position, and then the condyle and the disc slip in reverse of each other, resulting in incorrect relation between the disc and the condyle (Fig. **1**).

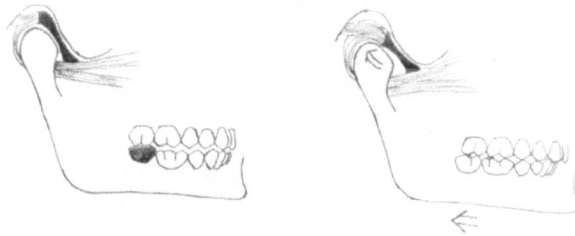

Figure 1: Mechanism of TMJ derangement.

In mandibular closure, the mandible moves posteriorly to meet multiple teeth from the muscular position to a more stable position (habitual occlusal position), and then the condyle and the disc slip in reverse, and the disc displacement occurs.

The correct relationship between the disc and the condyle is thought to be established fundamentally during the development of the functions of the masticatory muscles (with regard to the muscular position; that is the BPOP) before tooth eruption. Generally, tooth that erupt in a malposition that does not coincide with the centric relation may be correctly repositioned with the centric relation by muscular force; that is, the bite force. Under conditions in which an occlusal discrepancy exists until the tooth is repositioned into correct position, temporary clicking may be produced. However, if the bite force is small before the completion of the permanent dentition, the malposition of the occlusion will be maintained. Once the permanent dentition stage has been reached, usually at an age of 10-12 years, the muscles frequently adopt an occlusal position that does not coincide with the centric relation. This new position of occlusal contact usually begins as expedient process to avoid interferences, providing better function than the centric relation provides at that moment. The continued presence of the occlusal discrepancy causes the new reflex pattern of the pathway to be used so repeatedly that the new position of the mandible may resemble the centric relation. This acquired position can be regarded as the usual or habitual occlusal position (Moyers RE, 1956; Torii K, 2011). Rasmussen observed 119 patients in whom the progress of symptoms and radiographic abnormalities had been determined (Rasmussen OC, 1981). He divided temporomandibular arthropathy

(TMA) into six phases: Phases 1 and 2 make up an initial stage of clicking and locking, Phases 3 and 4 make up an intermediate stage of TMJ pain and constriction, and Phases 5 and 6 make up the terminal stage. Phase 5 is characterized by non-painful residual symptoms and Phase 6 by the complete disappearance of any subjective symptom. In control period, patients with lasting symptoms were followed from 1/2 to 5 1/2 years (Phase 5, 1st visit-Phase 5, control), and patients who recovered completely were followed from 1 to 5 years (Phase 6, 1st visit-Phase 6, control). He reported as follows: *In Phases 3 and 4* (intermediate stage), mandibular mobility was reduced (mean maximal opening 31-34 mm). In the TMJ affected, pain was present on maximal horizontal movement, more frequently on movement *from* (60-40%) rather than *to* (30-20%) the side of TMA. The capsule was tender to palpation in 75-60% of the patients, whereas crepitation was present in 25%. The opposite TMJ was intact in all patients. The masticatory muscles were tender in 50-70% of the patients on the side of TMA, and in 10-30% contralaterally (P<0.001). *In clinical Phase 4,* the lateral pterigoid muscle on the side of TMA was tender more frequently than the elevator muscles (P<0.05). *In clinical Phase 5*, mandibular mobility was slightly reduced. In the TMJ affected, pain was rarely present on maximal horizontal movement, whereas the capsule was tender in 10-15%. On the average, crepitation was present in 30% of the patients. However, a difference existed between patients with and without complete remission of symptoms. The contralateral TMJ was intact in all patients in Phase 5. The masticatory muscles were tender in 40% of the patients on the side of TMA, and in 10% contralaterally (P<0.001). *In clinical Phase 6*, mandibular mobility was normal. In the TMJ with arthropathy, capsular tenderness and crepitation were occasionally found. In the opposite TMJ clicking was found in 10% of the patients. The masticatory muscles were tender in 10-20% of the patients, without side difference and most often symmetrically. At the end of the *control period,* abnormality of the TMJs or masticatory muscles was found in 20-40% of the patients. Crepitation was found only on the side of TMA (25%), clicking was predominant contralaterally (10%), and muscular tenderness most often was bilateral (15%). All findings except crepitation and bilateral muscular tenderness improved in the course of Temporomandibular Arthropathy (TMA). In the case of maximal opening, improvement was significant between each of the phases, and the opening was normal in the terminal stage (44 mm). In the case of horizontal movement *from* the side of TMA, improvement took place among Phases 3, 4 and 5. Mobility *to* the side of TMA improved from Phase 3 to 4, and remained stable from then on. Tenderness of the TMJ capsule to palpation mainly improved from Phase 4 to 5, although some reduction took place from Phase 3 to 4. Tenderness of the arthropathic joint disappeared completely during the control period. Pain on maximal movement *from* and *to* the side of TMA mainly improved from Phase 4 to 5, although some reduction took place from Phase 3 to 4 in the case of movement *from*. TMJ pain on maximal horizontal movement disappeared completely during the control period. Crepitation generally remained unchanged in the course of TMA, although improvement tended to take place from Phase 5 to 6. However, patients with and without lasting symptoms differed with respect to the presence of crepitation. On the side of TMA, muscular tenderness, mainly improved from Phase 5 to 6. The elevators improved first from Phase 3 to 4 and the lateral pterigoid last from Phase 4 to 5. In the contralateral side, muscular tenderness improved from Phase 3 to 4 to remain stable from then on. From clinical Phase 5 and then on, patients with transient symptoms differed from patients with lasting residual symptoms. Crepitation was most frequently found in patients with lasting symptoms. Maximal opening was 4 mm larger in patients as compared to patients at the first visit in Phase 5. Pain on movement *from* the side of TMA and tenderness of the TMJ capsule and lateral pterigoid muscle tended to be most frequent in patients with lasting symptoms, whereas tenderness of the elevator muscles tended to be most frequent in patients with transient symptoms. On the side of TMA in patients with lasting symptoms, the lateral pterigoid muscle was more frequently tender than the elevator muscles, whereas these muscles were equally tender in patients becoming free from symptoms. In control period: *Patients with complete remission of symptoms*- After complete disappearance of symptoms, mandibular mobility still improved. Crepitation tended to improve from Phase 5 to 6, to become increasingly frequent during the control period. All other abnormal findings of the arthropathic TMJ disappeared. Tenderness of the lateral pterigoid muscle restricted to the side of TMA disappeared, whereas the bilateral tenderness of this muscle, as well as tenderness of the elevator muscles, remained unchanged during the control period, being present in 10-15% of these patients. In the contralateral TMJ clicking appeared in

10% of these patients in the transition from Phase 5 to 6. *Patients with lasting residual symptoms-* Crepitation became increasingly frequent, and was found in 60% of these patients at the end of the control period. Maximal opening increased by 2 mm. All other abnormal findings of the arthropathic TMJ improved or disappeared. Tenderness of the lateral pterigoid muscle on the affected side seemed to improve, whereas the elevators on this side, and all of the opposite muscles became increasingly and frequently tender during the control period. In neither group of patients was muscular atrophy found during the course of TMA or at the end of the control period. No abnormality by clinical examination was present in the contralateral TMJ in patients with lasting residual symptoms of TMA (Rasmussen OC, 1981). Rasmussen reports on the tenderness of elevator muscles show the existence of occlusal discrepancy between HOP (habitual occlusal position) and BPOP (bite plate-induced occlusal position), and imply that disk displacement of TMJ is caused by the occlusal discrepancy. Nickerson and Boering, observed 134 patients to find a correlation between condyle morphology on transpharyngeal radiographs and arthrographic diagnosis, pain, history of "locking", and interincisal opening (Nickerson JW & Boering G, 1989). They reported as follows: Fifty-four per cent of the 243 joints studied were painful. Ninety-eight per cent of these painful joints had an arthrographic diagnosis of ADR (anteriorly displaced disk with reduction) or ADNR (anteriorly displaced disk without reduction). Pain was least frequent when the condyle was deformed. This was most apparent when considered in association with ADNR 74% had pain with normal morphology, 69% had pain with small morphology, and 38% had pain with deformed morphology. Pain was most prominent in those with actively arthrotic morphology-90 per cent. Ninety-nine subjects had one joint with ADNR, and in 27 of these, both joints had ADNR. 65% of the patients had a history consistent to be progressed from clinical ADR to ADNR. They described as follows: Whatever the cause of disk displacement may be, it seems reasonable that the ligament attachment of the disk to the lateral pole, and at times to the medial pole, and the inferior lamina of the bilaminar zone must be enlongated. Whether this elongation is large the result of mechanical factors, systemic laxity of ligaments, a combination of these, or some other factors, remains to be elucidated. Only 37 per cent of Boering's patients went through what we recognized today clinically as a progression from ADR to ADNR and further went through an arthritic or an arthritic event. An "arthritic event" implies an inflammatory response producing pain during the osseous remodeling. The same remodeling can occur without pain, an "arthritic event". It has been documented that the arthritic or arthritic event "burns out", pain subsides, and the range of motion again becomes acceptable. This "burning out" refers to the course of the radiographycally demonstrable arthrotic event, and it makes no difference whether the arthrotic process appears soon after the disk becomes nonreducing or decays after the disk becomes nonreducing, or whether the arthrosis is considered a second or late arthritic event in a joint with a previous juvenile arthritic event. The ADR must progress to ADNR and an arthrotic event must occur for stabilization or burn-out to occur. By contrast, a painful joint associated with ADR, perhaps because of fibrosis of the bilaminar zone, became painless but remained an ADR, should be considered to have undergone "adaptation" rather than burn-out. If subsequently, the disk progressed to ADNR to be followed by an arthritic event, then the progress would be expected to burn-out at the end. It is clear that most reports on TMJ dysfunction do not include significant numbers of older patients, even though internal derangement is frequent in older individuals. The small propotion of older patients in the present study supports the concept that, rather than there being a process of relentless progression of pain and disability from TMJ internal derangement, the process usually becomes a relatively stable, symptomless condition in older people. It has been concluded that there is no evidence that a joint with anteriorly displaced disk with reduction (ADR) must progress to anteriorly displaced disk without reduction (ADNR), nor is there evidence that an arthritic reaction must develop in a joint with ADNR. As the individuals exist with internal derangements in all known stages without pain, the clinician is incorrect to assume, in a patient with pain and internal derangement, that the pain is necessarily the effect of the internal derangement.

An individual with an internal derangement with no pain may develop pain in future; however, the likelihood appears to diminish with age, especially after 40 years of age. Those who attempt to apply remedial treatments directed toward internal derangements must take into consideration that almost all forms of therapy are about 80 per cent successful, and the same degree of success may result from "natural" events (Nickerson JW & Boering G, 1989). However, if a patient with pain of ADR or ADNR, then he should be treated is present. In the case of ADR, it can be treated only with occlusal adjustment in the BPOP, or with a small restorations. However, in the case of ADNR, it will be treated with a large occlusal reconstruction, as described in Chapter 7. Therefore, it is advisable to treat ADR in early stage. ADNR is thought to be occurred with the enlongation of the ligament attachment of the disk by the backward displacement of condyle (Fig. **1**). Marguelles-Bonnet *et al.* compared the provisional diagnosis based on an initial clinical examination with subsequent findings of magnetic resonance imaging in patients with internal derangement of the TMJ. They reported that the magnetic resonance imaging and clinical diagnoses exactly matched in only 287 of the 484 joints studied, and the remaining 197 joints had only partial agreements. They described that degenerative arthrosis is a result of a long-term displaced disc (Marguelles-Bonnet RE *et al.*, 1995). Therefore, ADR or ADNR should not be left untreated.

SUMMARY

Although TMJ disc displacement with reduction will not necessarily progress to disc displacement without reduction, the TMJ clicking means the existence of the occlusal discrepancy. The existence of the occlusal discrepancy means potential pathological condition. Therefore, the occlusal discrepancy should be confirmed and corrected.

REFERENCES

Dao TTT, Lund JP, Lavigne GJ (1994). Pain responses to experimental chewing in myofascial pain paitents. *J Dent Res* 1994;73:1163-1167.

Fricton JR, Kroening R, Haley D, Siegert R (1985). Myofascial pain syndrome of the head and neck: A review of clinical characteristics of 164 patients. *Oral Surg Oral Med Ora Pathl* 1985;60:615-623.

Glaros AG, Tabacchi KN, Glass EG (1998). Effect of parafunctional clenching on TMD pain. *J Orofac Pain* 1998;12:145-152.

Mao J, Stein RB, Osborn JW (1993). Fatigue in human jaw muscles: a review. *J Orofac Pain* 1993;7:135-142.

McNamara JA, Seligman DA, Okeson JP (1995). Occlusion, orthodontic treatment, and temporomandibular disorders: A review. *J Orofac Pain* 1995;9:73-90.

Marguelles-Bonnet RE, Carpentier P, Yung JP, Defrennes D, Pharaboz C (1995). Clinical diagnosis compared with findings of magnetic resonance imaging in 242 patients with internal derangement of the TMJ. *J Orofac Pain* 1995;9:244-253.

Moyers RE (1956). Some physiologic considerations of centric and other jaw relations. *J Prosthet Dent* 1956;6:183-194.

Nickerson JW & Boering G (1989). Natural course of osteoarthrosis as it relates to internal derangement of the temporomandibular joint. *Oral Maxillofac Surg Clin North Am* 1989;1:27-45.

Obrez A & Stohler CS (1996). Jaw muscle pain and its effect on gothic arch tracings. *J Prosthet Dent* 1996;75:393-398.

Rasmussen OC (1981). Clinical findings during the course of temporomandibular arthropathy. *Scand J Dent Res* 1981;89:283-288.

Schwartz LL (1956). A temporomandibular joint pain dysfunction syndrome. *J Chronic Diseases* 1956;3:284-293.

Stohler CS (1999). Muscle-related temporomandibular disorders. *J Orofac Pain* 1999;13:273-284.

Svensson P & Graven-Nielsen T (2001). Craniofacial muscle pain: review of mechanisms and clinical manifestations. *J Orofac Pain* 2001;15:117-145.

Torii K & Chiwata I (2005). Relationship between habitual occlusal position and flat bite plane-induced occlusal position in volunteers with and without temporomandibular joint sounds. J Craniomandib Pract 2005;23:16-21.

Torii K & Chiwata I (2010). Occlusal adjustment using the bite plate-induced occlusal position as a reference position for temporomandibular disorders: a pilot study. *Head & Face Medicine* 2010,6:5. Available from: http://www.head-face-med.com/content/6/1/5

Toii k & Chiwata I (2010). A case report of the symptom-relieving action of an anterior flat plane bite plate for temporomandibular disorder. *The open Dentistry J* 2010;4:218-222. ISSN 1874-2106.

Torii K (2011). Longitudinal course of temporomandibular joint sounds in Japanese children and adolescents. *Head & Face Medicine* 2011, 7:17. Available from: http://www.head-face-med.com/7/1/17.

Send Orders for Reprints to reprints@benthamscience.net

CHAPTER 9

Various Symptoms of Temporomandibular Disorders

Abstract: Tension type headache is considered to manifest occur due to hypertension of masticatory muscles induced by occlusal discrepancy. Aural symptoms are also considered to occur due to hypertension of masticatory muscles or fatigue related to them. Burning mouth syndrome and glossodynia are considered to be caused by chorda tympani squeezed between malleus and incus.

Keywords: Tension type headache, burning mouth syndrome, glossodynia, facial pain, recurrent headache, clenching, TMJ pain dysfunction, muscle pain, stomatognathic treatment, migraine, muscle contraction headache, occlusal discrepancy, tinnitus, tensor tympani muscle, vertigo, otalgia, Ménière's disease.

1. INTRODUCTION

Patients with temporomandibular disorders (TMDs) complain of various symptoms besides facial pain, TMJ pain, and limitation of oral function. These symptoms include headache, aural symptoms, painful tongue (glossodynia) and burning sensation (burning mouth syndrome). The relation between headache and TMDs has been studied for a long time and the effectiveness of various treatments on headache has been evaluated.

2. HEADACHE

Recurrent headaches in relation to TMDs were investigated by Magnusson and Carlsson (Mafnusson T & Carlsson GE, 1978). They reported that clenching of teeth was correlated to the severity of headache. The frequency and severity of headache varied also with the severity of TMD. Of the variables included in the dysfunction index, only masticatory musculature painful to palpation was found to have a distinct relationship with headache. They described that functional treatment is indicated in patients with headaches and tenderness of the masticatory musculature, which is elaborated as follows: A correlation between frequency of headache and functional disturbances of the masticatory system has been shown by many authors, as it has been highlighted in the present study. This investigation also showed a significant correlation between the patient's opinion of the severity of headache and the degree of clinically recorded TMJ pain-dysfunction. The correlation with TMJ pain-dysfunction remained unchanged when the severity of headache was added to the frequency of the symptom. This may be explained by the assumption that the patient's opinion of the severity of headache is substantially influenced by the frequency of the symptom, *i.e.,* there is a close covariation between the patient's opinion of the severity and the frequency of headache. There was a correlation between TMJ pain and headaches, but only in combination with muscle pain. When the influence of muscle pain was eliminated, the correlation was no longer identifiable. Of the components of dysfunction index, tenderness of the masticatory musculature to palpation was thus the most reliable indicator of headaches being related to functional disturbances of the masticatory system. Also, tenderness of the temporalis has been found to be associated with muscular hyperactivity. Tension and hyperactivity of the muscles in the face and the head can contribute both to tension headache and to functional disturbances of the masticatory system. In addition, Magnusson and Carlsson compared the effect of stomatognathic treatment (occlusal splint, occlusal adjustment, and exercise therapy) and the conventional dental treatment on headache (Magnusson T & Carlsson GE, 1980). They concluded that the stomatognathic treatment has a beneficial effect on TMDs and many patients who suffer recurrent headaches experience a reduction in the frequency and severity of their headaches after the treatment. Forssell *et al.,* also reported that the frequency of headache was reduced in 79% and intensity in 53% of patients suffering from muscle contraction headache or combination headache in whom the adjustment of dental occlusion had been successfully accomplished. They defined that occlusal treatment of pure migraine did not prove superior to placebo treatment. Our previous studies seemed to indicate that muscle tension could be associated with migraine headache. However, the present study did not give any clues about the possible primary role of muscle tension in the pain mechanisms of migraine. In contrast to pure migraine, combination headache patients responded favorably to the treatment of mandibular dysfunction. The effect of treatment on muscle contraction headache was significantly better than that of the placebo treatment. Both the frequency and intensity of headache were reduced (Forssell H *et al.,* 1985). Karppinen *et al.,* also reported that short term response to therapy was good in both groups (occlusal adjustment group and a mock adjustment group), however, in the long-term, the response was significantly better in patients who had undergone occlusal adjustment than in the mock adjusted controls (Karppinen K *et al.*, 1999). However, Forssell *et al.,* concluded that evidence of the use of occlusal adjustment is lacking (Forssell H *et al.*, 1999; Forssell H & Kalso E, 2004)). As previously described in Chapter 3 and 4, their occlusal adjustment used the reference position of retruded contact position, and the effectiveness of this procedure has not been demonstrated. Svensson described that patients with tension-type headache and migraine will more frequently develop headache following sustained tooth-clenching than will healthy control subjects (Svensson P, & Graven-Nielsen T, 2001). There is always a possibility of tension-type headache to occur, because higher activity of masticatory muscles in TMD patients than those of subjects without TMD is induced with the occlusal discrepancy between HOP and BPOP. Elimination of the occlusal discrepancy by occlusal equilibration resolves tension-type headache. Our treatment outcome for headache will be described in Chapter 10. The occlusal adjustment performed in the reference position of the muscular contact position was very effective for headache, especially in patients with myofascial pain.

3. AURAL SYMPTOMS

The first description of the relationship between TMJ dysfunction and aural symptoms is thought to have been made by Costen in 1934. Costen reported various clinical cases of patients with ear and nasal symptoms; he summarized his findings stating that hearing tests showed a mild type of catarrhal otitis with the involvement of Eustachian tube (usually simple obstruction). The prognosis of such cases repeatedly depended on these factors: (a) the accuracy with which refitted dentures relieved the abnormal pressure on the joint; and (b) the extent of the injury to the tube condyle, meniscus and joint capsule (Costen JB, 1934, 1936, 1944). However, Sicher reported that from an anatomical perspective, the Eustachian tube could not be compressed during the closure of the mandible; neither can the opening action of the tensor palate muscle on the tube could not be impaired in this condition, making Costen's theory impossible (Sicher H, 1948). Schwartz theorized that contractive muscle spasm may cause pain as a direct result of myofascial trigger mechanism by referred routes (Schwartz LL, 1956). Dolowitz *et al.*, reported that muscle exercises were effective for the relief of aural symptoms, especially ear fullness and tinnitus. Various therapies have since been tried for the relief of TMD symptoms, including aural symptoms (Dolowitz DA *et al.*, 1964). These therapies include selective grinding of the teeth, bite plate, biofeedback training, thermotherapy and muscle training (Koskinnen J *et al.*, 1980; Principato JJ & Barwell DR, 1978). Erlandsson *et al.*, reported that stomatognathic treatment (occlusal adjustment, occlusal splint, and exercise therapy) and biofeedback treatment seem to have some positive effects on a subgroup of tinnitus patients (with normal hearing) (Erlandsson SI *et al.*, 1991). Rubinstein performed extensive studies of TMD and tinnitus and made the following conclusions: (1) 46% of the patients who received stomatognathic treatment reported no tinnitus or reduced tinnitus a few months after treatment. A two-year follow-up showed that the improvement persisted in most of those who had benefited from the treatment. (2) Frequent headaches, fatigue/tenderness in the jaw muscles, clinical findings of pain upon palpation of the masticatory muscles, impaired mandibular mobility, and signs of parafunctions were more prevalent among tinnitus patients than among an epidemiological sampling. (3) The awareness of diurnal bruxism and a feeling of jaw tenderness/fatigue may be related to fluctuating tinnitus, vertigo and hyperacusis. (4) The evaluation of treatment outcome showed some improvements at the group level: a decrease in tinnitus, mood improvement, and a reduction in clinical signs of the dysfunction of the masticatory system. (5) A strong relationship existed between tinnitus complaints and several symptoms of TMD. In summary, a relatively low severity of tinnitus, normal hearing, and fluctuations in the tinnitus intensity were good predictors of the psychological, stomatognathic and cervical treatment outcome (Rubinstein B, 1993). Chan and Reade reported that tinnitus may have a multifactorial etiology, similar to pain, for which the correction or elimination of any one of the factors may result in the complete resolution of symptoms (Chan SWY & Riede PC, 1994). Thus, the absence of any significant or detectable auditory, genetic, drug-related, or trauma-related causes should be confirmed by otolaryngologists before treating TMD patients with tinnitus. Myrhaug observed many patients who sought help because of neuralgic type pains of the face, headache and temporomandibular arthrosis resulting from bite anomalies. He described that bite anomalies regularly lead to tensions and contraction states in the masticatory muscles which can be demonstrated by electromyography. On a similar basis, the two tensor muscles (tensor tympani and tensor veli palatine) also influenced through their common nerve supply (nervus trigeminus). This has been demonstrated visually during operations for otosclerosis when the drum head is reflected. Contractions of the tensor tympani muscle can be observed directly under the operating microscope when stimulated voluntarily by grinning and clenching movements of the jaw. By contraction of the tensor tympani muscle, the shaft of the hammer is pulled inward and foreshortened. This can be seen regularly when there is a state of tension in the muscles innervated by the trigeminal nerve as a consequence of bite anomalies. It is mentioned by otologists that bite deformity is a known cause of tinnitus aurium. The sound that the patient hears, is not due to external sound wave as in the usual hearing reaction. This tinnitus arises as an autogenous vibration in the sound-conducting system, and it seems to be due to tremor or myoclonus (myorhythmia) in the tensor muscle of the middle ear. It represents a fatigue reaction resulting from prolonged irritation and stress of the muscles innervated by the trigeminal nerve (masticators). This form of fatigue reaction apparently only affects the small muscles in this group because of its anatomical relationship. Hence, the two tensor muscles are in a vulnerable position in bite anomalies. There may, also, be autophony, a condition in which one hears one's voice inside the head as if speaking into an empty barrel. In such cases, there is contraction (spasm) in the tensor muscle of the soft palate causing fullness in the ear and temporary deafness. It is relevant in the explanation of the vestibular type of vertigo that the violent dizzy attacks generally start with strong and intense tinnitus and are often associated with headache. It is suggested that such attacks can arise from sudden and severe movements of the footplate of the stapes. A ripple of the waves arises in the lymph of the inner ear, which gives rise to these reactions and exerts an intermittent pressure on the walls of the labyrinth. This is similar to the waves breaking on the shore. The hollowing out of the labyrinth found in Ménière's disease, called 'hydrops', may be well explained as the result of such pressure effects as no real increase of pressure in the labyrinth has been measured. By removing the causative factors which can be done by adequate restoration of the bite, the attacks can be checked and the subjective ear symptoms reduced or brought to an end. The issue here is an oto-dental syndrome which demands close co-operation between medical and dental practitioner (Myrhaug H, 1964-1965). Koskinnen *et al.*, and Parker and Chole were skeptical about Myrhaug's theory (Koskinnen J *et al.*, 1980; Parker ES & Chole RA, 1995). However, Watanabe *et al.*, reported that tinnitus occurred whenever a certain mimic facial muscle contracted voluntarily or involuntarily. Under the operating microscope, the contraction of the stapedial muscle synchronous with the contraction of the mimic facial muscle was observed. The tinnitus disappeared completely immediately after the tendon of the stapedial muscle was sectioned (Watanabe I *et al.*, 1974). Lam *et al.*, investigated TMD patients regarding aural symptoms, and reported that of the 344 subjects with TMD, 59.9% complained of aural symptoms, as against 29.2% of the 432 patients without TMD. Of the subjects with otalgia, tinnitus, vertigo, or perceived hearing loss, 67%, 64.1%, 65.2%, and 62.2% respectively had TMD. In addition, they described that when compared to the non-aural symptoms group, the subjects with aural symptoms more often had masticatory muscles that were tender to palpation. Lam *et al.,* described that Kuttila *et al.,* also repoted that subjects with aural symptoms had more clinical signs of TMD, such as pain on palpation of TMJs or masticatory muscles. It would have been interesting to compare the intensity of muscular pain with that of the aural symptoms; however, the severity of aural symptoms was not estimated in our study (Lam DK *et al.*, 2001) or in that of Kuttila *et al.,* (Kuttila S *et al.*, 1999). They also described that the potential for clinician bias on patients' reports of referred pain was not estimated in these studies. A recent study has found that bias induced by instructions from the clinician can result in an over-report of the presence and intensity of referred pain upon muscle palpation in TMD patients. The study indicated that factors such as the patients' attention, their expectations, and their level of anxiety or response bias affected pain report. Thus, in an effort to reduce clinician bias, the 4 clinicians who worked on this study consistently relied on the standardized histories and examination forms when making their assessments of patients' pain reports throughout the 12 years of the study. Our study also found that patients with dental percussion sensitivity were more likely to suffer from aural symptoms. This association may be related to a central trigeminal connection linking oral pain with aural pain, although it is not entirely clear how the local neural network in the TMJ region sends afferent nociceptive input to cortical areas of the brain. Moreover, dental percussion causes vibrations similar to those caused by the mechanics of stomatognathic system during oral function, and these vibrations of a dental origin are conducted most effectively to the ear (dentaural hearing). It should also be noted that patients with TMD have the propensity for referred craniofacial pain; this might explain the findings in the present study of a significantly greater frequency of aural complaints in TMD than in non-TMD pain conditions. Referred aural pain is prevalent in the craniofacial region, as reported in a recent retrospective study of patients with TMD. The greater frequency of aural complaints in TMD *versus* non-TMD pain conditions is significant because it suggests the possibility that TMD nociceptive mechnisms differ from those of other craniofacial pain conditions. There may be differences in the primary nociceptive afferents innervating the TMJ (capsule, disc, and associated musculature) or in the relay and processing of noxious stimuli in the spinal nucleus of the trigeminal nerve, particularly the subnucleus caudalis, in terms of nociceptive receptors and/or mediators. Clearly, further study of the nociceptive mechanisms involved in TMD pain is necessary. Likewise, clinical trials of TMD therapies would also aid in establishing a cause-and-effect relationship. Such evidence may help individuals suffering from ear symptoms to isolate the cause of their symptoms and also preclude the need for unnecessary otologic surgical procedures (Lam DK *et al.*, 2001). Torii described that taking into account the facts that myofascial pain, disc displacement, tension-type headaches and tinnitus were resolved after occlusal equilibrating treatment in the BPOP, tinnitus related to TMD may be caused by the spasmodic synkinesis of the tensor tympani and the stapedial muscle with muscle spasm of the masticatory muscles (including relative muscles), or by a decrease in the blood supply to the middle and inner ear with noxious stimuli to the peridiscal tissue, or by increased endolymphatic pressure with injury to the peridiscal tissues of the TMJ (Torii K, 2011). The following is a case of a patient with aural symptoms together with the occlusal discrepancy between the HOP and BPOP (Torii K & Chiwata I, 2007): A 73-year old woman presented with the chief complaint of severe pain and tinnitus in the right ear. She reported that while performing karaoke 2 years back, she suddenly felt a strong impact on her right ear and developed such a severe rotatory vertigo that she was unable to stand and had to crawl on the floor. She was diagnosed with Ménièr's disease by two independent otorhinolaryngologists and was treated with isosorbide, mecobalamin and ibudilast. However, when the drugs failed to improve her severe symptoms, she came to our clinic. The patient's medical history was unremarkable. No impairment of mouth opening, no deviation of the opening path, and no noises in either of the TMJs were detected. The patient reported tenderness on palpation of the right TMJ and tenderness of the right lateral pterygoid muscle. Twenty-nine teeth were present, and the upper right third molar was slightly extruded because there was no opposing tooth. Occlusion was anatomically normal. The right TMJ appeared unclear on the TMJ computed tomography (CT) images in the HOP from the first consultation. The cause of the lack of clarity was unknown, but it seemed to be attributable to inflammation, or to the eccentricity of the condyle in the glenoid fossa. For this patient, three HOP records were obtained by voluntary jaw closing at the first visit. Since an anterior flat plane bite plate was recommended as a provisional appliance to decrease painful symptoms, an anterior flat plane bite plate was directly fabricated in the patient's mouth using self-curing acrylic resin, which the patient wore every night for a week. At the second visit (one week after the first visit), her otalgia had ceased, and the intensity of the tinnitus was greatly diminished. The BPOP records were obtained during voluntary jaw closing, in the upright position and after wearing the bite plate for five minutes. To examine the difference between the HOP and BPOP, three-dimensional measurements were performed on the modified articulator using previous records. The shift from the HOP to BPOP was significant, using ANOVA for a two factor experiment with repeated measurements for both position factors ($p<0.005$).

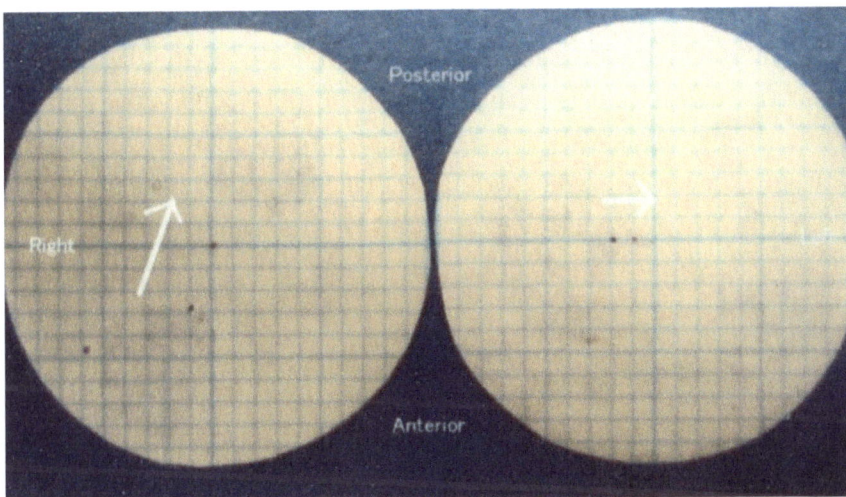

Figure 1: The shift from HOP to BPOP recorded on both condylar areas of the articulator.

The degree of the shift indicates the actual change in the patient's condyle because the inter- condylar distance of the articulator was adjusted to the same distance as that of the patient. The white arrow indicates the shift from the HOP to the BPOP.

In the present case, extraction of the right upper third molar was selected first, because of premature occlusal contact in the BPOP. Subsequently, occlusal adjustment in the BPOP was performed 5 times during 2 months. At the completion of the occlusal adjustment, the difference between the HOP and BPOP was not significant (p>0.25), and the right condyle shifted 2.8 mm posteromedially in the horizontal plane, and the left condyle shifted 1.0 mm laterally from the previously recorded HOP (Fig. **1**). The patient's aural symptoms completely resolved, and no recurrence has been reported in symptoms and reappearance of the discrepancy between the HOP and BPOP to date after a 7-year follow-up period. The outcome of occlusal adjustment in the muscular contact position for aural symptoms of patients with TMD will be shown in Chapter 10.

4. BURNING MOUTH SYNDROME AND GLOSSODYNIA

Burning mouth syndrome (BMS) is characterized by burning and painful sensations in clinically normal oral mucosa. Cibirka *et al.,* described various etiologies: Local factors: (1) Dental treatment (The onset of symptoms, as reported by patients related to previous dental treatment, may be as high as 65%.); (2) Infectious agents (Candidiasis has been the most frequently identified infectious agent.); (3) Allergic reaction (Mucosal allergic reactions to allergens such as methyl methacrylate monomer and nickel sulfate.); (4) Dysfunction and parafunction (Dysfunction and parafunction have been documented as frequent causative factors.); Quantity and quality of saliva (Inadequate saliva or dry mouth; Irregularities of saliva metabolites); and (5) Neural mechanism (Nerve injury or dysfunction resulting from oral, facial, or systemic trauma from medical conditions might be the cause of burning mouth syndrome) Systemic factors: Deficiency disease, hormonal and immunologic disturbances, and pharmacotherapuetic side effects have been implicated; Psychogenic factors comprise of: Depression, being noted as the next most important etiologic factor. The multiple etiologic factors for diagnosis of BMS present a challenging scenario for the dental clinician. Generally, the normal appearing mucosa, coupled with variable symptoms of oral pain, offers a formidable task for definitive diagnosis. Identification of the etiologic group, local, systemic, or psychogenic, will provide initial direction toward a diagnostic and treatment course. Dental or infectious origins may require intervention by the clinician. Advise and control of parafunctional activity, identification of salivary imbalances, prosthesis adjustment, or pharmacotherapuetic management may be indicated. Pharmacotherapuetics may empirically be used to achieve resolution for infectious agents or provide palliation of symptoms. Symptomatic relief may be achieved by rinsing with Benadryl elixir (Park-Davis, Morris Plains, N.J.) (12.5 mg/5 ml), 1 teaspoonful for 2 minutes before meals and swallowing; or a suspension of 30 ml Mycostatin (Apothecon, Princeton, N.J.) (100,000 units/ml), 50 ml hydrocortisone (10mg/5ml), 60 ml tetracycline (125 mg/5 ml) and 120 ml Benadryl elixir (12.5 mg/5 ml), 1 teaspoonful orally four times per day and expectorate. Allergic testing of materials, foods, or additives may be supportive in diagnosis and management. Evaluation by an oral pathologist may be helpful. Occasionally, otolaryngology and gastroenterology consultation may assist diagnosis of pharyngeal, esophageal, or reflux-related causes and provide medical care. Systemic factors usually require medical assistance for the correlation of imbalances in the oral symptoms described. Familiarization of the physician to documented correlations of oral symptoms to medical conditions may be necessary. Blood sera analysis, immunologic, or endocrine assessment may be required. Psychological consultation or psychological support may be helpful in diagnosis and care of the patient with BMS (Cibirka RM *et al.*, 1997). Danhauer *et al.*, compared burning mouth syndrome (BMS) and oral burning (OB) resulting from other clinical abnormatities. They reported the following Significant differences were not noted between groups for pain duration (in year); age; number of systemic illnesses; number of involved pain sites; number of teeth either decayed, missing, or filled; current smoking status; presence of an instigating event; perceived taste disturbance; perceived oral dryness; use of angiotensin-converting enzyme (ACE) inhibitors; anemia; geographic tongue; diabetes/abnormal glucose; and presence of fungal infection (P>.05). Participants with OB demonstrated more clinical abnormalities (46.55% of OB group *versus* 0% of BMS group, x^2 = 17.03, P<.001); hyposalivation (44.2% of OB group *versus* 0% of BMS group, x^2 = 16.22, P<.001); and greater use of prescription medications (mean = 4.35 prescriptions, SD = 3.58 for OB group; mean = 2.19 prescriptions, SD =3.16 for BMS group; *t*-test = -2.50, P<.05). Most notably, hormone replacement therapy was more common in the OB as group compared to the BMS group (39.5% of OB group *versus* 11.5% of BMS group, x^2 =6.17, P<.05). Clinical outcome was based on follow up of all subjects for a minimum period of 6 months. For the OB group, the mean follow-up period was 11.2 months (range 6 to 47 months). In the BMS group, the mean follow-up period was 10.5 months (range 6 to 48 months). When treatment was provided that corrected an identifiable abnormality, significantly (P<.05) more OB than BMS participants reported greater than 50% relief from the symptoms (72.5% *versus* 41.2%, respectively). The majority of BMS participants who were treated with norpramine and/or clonazepam, as described, reported a significant decrease in the symptoms. Complete relief was gained with 3 agents (*i.e.* norpramine, oxygen, and carbamazepine). The response to norpramine occurred generally at a low dose (less than 30 mg) and was seldom found to provide a benefit at doses greater than 50 mg. Oxgen was provided in an office setting at 100% and 4 to 5 L/minute. The beneficial effect of clonazepam was similar to previous findings, with no patient reporting complete relief. They concluded that while BMS and OB groups may initially present with similar clinical and psychosocial features, they are distinguishable with caerful diagnosis that often enables successful management of symptoms for each group (Danhauer SC *et al.*, 2002). Zakrzewska *et al.*, performed a systemic review of interventions for the treatment of burning mouth syndrome and they reported that none of the trials were able to provide conclusive evidence of effectiveness. However, cognitive behavioral therapy may be beneficial in reducing the intensity of the symptoms. They concluded that given that the research evidence is, as yet, unable to provide clear, conclusive evidence of an effective intervention, clinicians need to provide support and understanding when dealing with BMS sufferers. Psychological interventions that help patients to cope with symptoms may be of some use, but promising and new approaches to treatment still need to be evaluated in good-quality randomized controlled trials (Zakrzewska JM *et al.*, 2003). The following is a case of a patient with burning mouth syndrome: A twenty-five-year old woman presented with a chief complaint of burning sensations on palatal mucosa and the dorsum linguae. She reported that she felt pain on her tongue five months back, and visited an otorhinolaryngologic clinic and was she prescribed a gargle, but the drug failed to improve her severe symptoms, and then visited us. The patient's medical history was unremarkable. Twenty-eight teeth were present, and occlusion was anatomically normal. To examine the functional occlusal relationship between upper and lower jaws, an anterior flat bite plate was directly fabricated in the mouth and an occlusal analysis was performed on casts mounted on an articulator with the BPOP wax record. The premature occlusal contacts were located on both second molars, and then on the first molars after removing the contact on the second molars. A total of 11 occlusal adjustments in the BPOP were performed to obtain the occlusal contacts on both premolar and molar regions during five months. After that, the symptoms completely disappeared and no recurrence has been reported to date after a seven-year follow-up period. The author experienced several patients with glossodynia and their symptoms resolved with similar occlusal adjustment in the BPOP. Myrhaug described that the compression of the chain of ear bones which one must, also, presume to exist with the retraction of the tympanic membrane, may lead to contusion of the chorda tympani in its course between the hammer and the anvil (Fig. **2**). This anatomical relationship has not been previously connected with glossodynia, that smarting and burning sensation in the tongue is usually unilateral and has been observed many times to clear up after correction of bite defects. It is quite likely that there is a causal relationship here (Myrhaug H, 1964-1965).

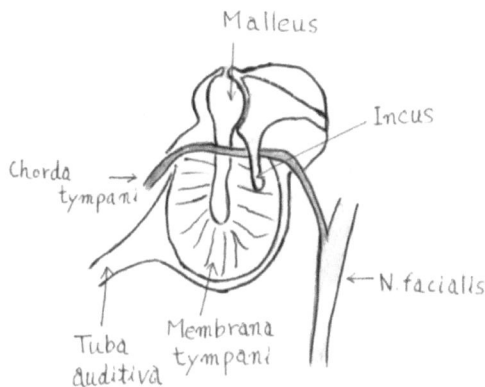

Figure 2: The relationship between Chorda tympani and Malleus and Incus.

When a patient presents with any of the symptoms mentioned above, he/she should not be given assurance that the symptom will be resolved. Initially an examination of patient's occlusion on dental casts mounted on an articulator must be performed, and if any premature contact is recognized on the casts, the occlusion is corrected. If the symptom have disappears after the adjustment is completed, the patient is fortunate. However, the symptom persists, the patient should be recommend to seek any clinical division any premature contact is not recognized.

SUMMARY

It is important to suspect a cause in occlusion, because imbalance of occlusion in the muscular contact position is thought to cause in any pathological conditions.

REFERENCES

Chan SEY & Riede PC (1994). Tinnitus and temporomandibular pain-dysfunction disorder. *Clin Otolaryngol Aliied Sci* 1994;19:370-380.

Cibirka RM, Nelson SK, Lefebvre CA (1997). Burning mouth syndrome: A review of etiologies. *J Prosthet Dent* 1997:78:93-97.

Costen JB (1934). A syndrome of ear and sinus symptoms dependent upon disturbed function of the temporomandibular joint. *Ann Otol Rhinol and Laryngol* 1934;43:1-15.

Costen JB (1936). Neuralgias and ear symptoms; associated with disturbed function of the temporomandibular joint. *JAMA* 1936;107:252-255.

Costen JB (1944). Diagnosis of mandibular joint neuralgia and its place in general head pain. *Ann Otol Rhinol and Laryngol* 1944;53:655-659.

Danhauer SC, MillerCS, Rhodus NL, Carlson CR (2002). Impact of criteria-based diagnosis of burning mouth syndrome on treatment outcome. *J Orofac Pain* 2002;16:305-311.

Dolowitz DA, Ward JW, Fingerle CO, Smith CC (1964). The role of muscular incoordination in the pathogenesis of temporomandibular joint syndrome. *Laryngoscope* 1964;74:790-801.

Erlandsson SI, Rubinstein B, Carlsson SG (1991). Tinnitus : evaluation of biofeedback and stomaognathic treatment. *Brit J Audiol* 1991;25:151-161.

Forssell H, Kirveskari P, Kangasniemi P (1985). Changes in headache after treatment of mandibular dysfunction. *Cephalalgia* 1985;5:229-236.

Forssell H, Kalso E, Koskela P Vehmanen R, Puukka P, Alanen P (1999). Occlusal treatments in temporomandibular disorders: a qualitative systemic review of randomized controlled trials.*Pain* 1999;83:549-560.

Forssell H & Kalso E (2004). Application of principles of evidence-based medicine to occlusal treatment for temporomandibular disorders: Are there lessons to be learned? *J Orofac Pain* 2004;18:9-22.

Karppinen K, Eklund S, Suoninen E Eskelin M Kirveskari P (1999). Adjustment of dental occlusion in treatment of chronic cervicobrachial pain and headache. *J Oral Rehabil* 1999;26:715-721.

Koskinnen J, Paavolainen M, Raivio M, Roschier J (1980). Otological manifestations in temporomandibular joint dysfunction. *J Oral Rehabil* 1980;7:249-254.

Kuttila S, Kuttila M, Le Bell Y, Alanen P (1999). Aural symptoms and signs of temporomandibular disorder in association with treatment need and visits to a physician. *Laryngoscope* 1999;109:1669-1673.

Lam DK, Lawrence HP, Tenenbaum HC (2001). Aural symptoms in temporomandibular disorder patients attending a craniofacial pain unit. *J Orofac Pain* 2001;15:146-157.

Magnusson T & Carlsson GE (1978). Recurrent headaches in relation to temporomandibular joint pain-dysfunction. *Acta Odontol Scand* 1978;36:333-338.

Magnusson T & Carlsson GE (1980). Changes in recurrent headaches and mandibular dysfunction after various types of dental treatment. *Acta Odontol Scand* 1980;38:311-320.

Myrhaug H (1964-1965). The incidence of ear symptoms in cases of malocclusion and temporomandibualr joint disturbances. *Br J Oral Surg* 1964-1965;2:28-32.

Parker WS & Chole RA (1995). Tinnitus, vertigo, and temporomandibualr disorders. *Am J Orthod Dentofac Orthop* 1995;107:153-158.

Principato JJ & Barwell DR (1978). Biofeedback training and relaxation exercises for treatment of temporomandibular joint dysfunction. *Otolaryngology* 1978;86:766-769.

Rubinstein B (1993). Tinnitus and craniomandibualr disorders: Is there a link? *Swed Dent J* 1993;95(Suppl):1-46.

Sicher H (1948). Temporomandibualr articulation in mandibular over-closure. *J Am Dent Assoc* 1948;36:131-139.

Svensson P & Graven-Nielsen T (2001). Craniofacial muscle pain: Review of mechanism and clinical manifestations. *J Orofac Pain* 2001;15:117-145.

Torii K & Chiwata I (2007). Occlusal management for a patient with aural symptoms of unknown etiology: a case report. *J Med Case Rep* 2007,1:85. Available from: http://www.jmedicalcasereports.com/content/1/1/85

Torii K. (2011). Tinnitus and temporomandibular disorders, In: *Up to Date on Tinnitus,* Fayez Bahmad Jr, pp. (17), InTech, Available from: www.intechopen.com

Watanabe I, Kumagami H, Tsuda Y (1974). Tinnitus due to abnormal contraction of stapedial muscle. An abnormal phenomenon in the course of facial nerve paralysis and its audiological significance. *ORL* 1974;36:217-226.

Zakrzewska JM, Forssell H, Glenny A (2003). Interventions for the treatment of burning mouth syndrome: A systematic review. *J Orofac Pain* 2003;17:293-300.

CHAPTER 10

Treatment Outcome of Temporomandibualr Disorders

Abstract: Conservative treatments for temporomandibular disorders (TMDs) are symptomatic treatments, and therefore, they cannot completely cure TMDs. The signs and symptoms of TMDs completely disappear by using occlusal equilibration in the muscular contact position (MCP). This is a causal treatment for TMDs. The evaluation of outcome of treatment should be performed to strictly confirm whether or not signs and symptoms have disappeared.

Keywords: Conservative treatment, causal treatment, invasive treatment, occlusal adjustment, prosthetic treatment, disc dislocation, arthrogenous problem, myogenous problem, myofascial pain syndrome, medication, biofeedback, relaxation training, transcutaneous nerve stimulation, psychologic counseling, prosthesis, retruded contact position.

1. INTRODUCTION

It is difficult to compare the treatment outcome of temporomandibular disorders (TMDs) in studies that have been performed until date, because the treatment modality varied in those studies or various modalities were included in one study. However, the treatment outcomes may be divided into the outcome from invasive treatment and conservative treatment. Since the treatment outcome from occlusal adjustment using the retruded contact position (RCP) as a reference position has not been demonstrated to be effective for TMD, conservative treatment is recommended for TMDs at present.

2. OUTCOME OF CONSERVATIVE TREATMENT

De Boever *et al.* compared treatment outcomes of an elderly and a younger TMD group. They described that one would expect a higher prevalence of older patients with a joint disorder. Only 4 of 68 elderly patients were diagnosed with polyarthritis involving the TMJ. It is likely that the elderly patients take more analgesics and tranquilizers for facial pain problems instead of seeking treatment. However, a large group of elderly patients with general joint diseases that involve the TMJ were referred to the Facial Pain Unit for adequate and proper conservative treatment in addition to general therapy. They concluded as follows: 1) Patients over 50 years of age represented only 21% of patients who had temporomandibualr pain and dysfunction diagnosed and who received treatment in the Facial Pain Unit over the test period, despite the increase of general joint diseases in the elderly. 2) The younger patient group between 20 and 30 years of age and the older group between 50 and 70 years of age differed in a higher pain level, more general disorders, and medication in the latter group and greater pain in the joints in the first group. 3) Other clinical signs, such as pain in the muscles, duration of symptoms, maximal mouth opening capacity, and even distribution of temporomandibular disorder diagnoses were not different. 4) Both groups responded equally well to a conservative treatment regimen that resulted in a marked reduction of pain and dysfunction. However, some forms of occlusal therapy (occlusal equilibration, prosthetic treatment) were included in their study. They reported that 1 case of disc dislocation in group I (young group) was in a worse condition after 1 year. In group II (older group), 4 patients worsened during the year despite therapy; 1 patient experienced rheumatoid arthritis; had mainly myogenous problems; and 1 patient was diagnosed with a combined arthrogenous/myogenous problem (De Boever JA *et al.*, 1999). These patients with severe symptoms were rare, but they were in serious problem. Green & Laskin investigated the effect of treatment on myofascial pain syndrome (MPD). They highlighted that the subjects of this study included 175 patients with MPD who had been treated at the Temporomandibular Joint and Facial Pain Research Center. Patients with TMJ clicking and other minor movement disorders that are currently labeled as internal derangements were included in this population, but patients with major movement disorders recurrent dislocation, "closed lock", were excluded after. At least one year had passed since treatment was concluded, and in some cases as long as 11 years had elapsed, the mean was about five years. The study data were obtained from telephone interviews that were conducted by research assistants under the supervision of Dr. Greene. A wide variety of treatments were used during the 11 years in which these patients were treated. The treatment modalities used during this period included various medications, oral appliances, biofeedback, relaxation training, mock-equilibration, transcutaneous nerve stimulation, and psychological counseling. The common factor among them was their reversibility of action; none produced permanent changes in dental morphology or in craniomandibular relationships. In addition, these treatments generally required some degree of cooperation and participation from the patients in order to be maximally effective. When they were charged from the center, all successfully treated patients were advised about self-management techniques, including some based on their particular therapy and some on general principles such as limitations in diet, restrictions in movement, and application of heat. It should be emphasized that patients who, by chance received placebo treatments were never informed of this fact, and they were charged in the same manner as other patients. An analysis of the clinical records of the 175 patients in this study disclosed that 130 (74%) were greatly improved or totally free of symptoms when they were charged from the center. Forty-three patients (25%) showed only minor or no improvement when they were charged, and two (1%) became worse during therapy. During the telephone interviews, it was found that 42 patients had sought further professional treatment after leaving the center. Of these, 24 (57%) reported improvement of their symptoms after further treatment, and 18 (43%) reported no improvement. However, about half of the patients in the latter subgroup of nonresponders reported that gradual improvement occurred after they discontinued all forms of professional therapy. Ninety per cent of the patients reported that they were doing well, with 53% describing themselves as asymptomatic, and 37% experiencing only minor residual or recurrent symptoms. Only 8% regarded themselves as essentially unimproved, and 2% thought that their symptoms were currently worse than when they first came to the center. Green and Laskin highlighted that these results were compared with those from ten published papers in which investigators used either irreversible treatment methods, reversible methods, or a combination of both approaches. The treatment outcome results in this study were similar to those in all of the previously reported studies. These findings suggest that conservative reversible therapies are both sufficient and appropriate for the management of MPD syndrome in most patients. Major alterations of mandibular position or dentoalveolar relationships do not appear to be necessary for obtaining either short-term or long-term success, and therefore, they can be generally regarded as an inappropriate treatment for this disorder (Green CS & Laskin DM, 1983). However, their data were obtained from telephone interview and the patients were not clinically examined after treatment. In addition, the patients with severe symptoms were excluded. Several patients were worse similar the study of De Boever *et al.* Ekberg *et al.* observed the efficacy of appliance therapy, and reported that the stabilization appliance was more effective in alleviating symptoms and signs in patients with TMD of mainly myogenous origin than a control, non-occlusal appliance in short-term evaluation (Ekberg E, 2003). However, signs such as muscle tenderness and TMJ tenderness did not mostly change after appliance therapy. Schmitter *et al.* performed a comparative evaluation of different types of splint therapy for anterior disc displacement without reduction (ADDWR) of temporomandibular joint and indicated that: 38 patients received a centric splint, while 36 received a distraction splint, randomly. After 1, 3, and 6 months of therapy, outcome was evaluated using the Wilcoxon signed rank test for matched pairs. Success after 6 months was defined as an improvement in active mouth opening of more than 20% patients and pain reduction (on chewing) of at least 50%. They reported that centric splints seem to be more effective than distraction splints for ADDWR (Schmitter M *et al.*, 2005). Truelove *et al.* randomized 200 subjects diagnosed with TMD into three groups: usual conservative, dentist-prescribed self-care treatment without any intraoral appliance (UT); UT plus a conventional flat-plane hard acrylic splint (HS); and UT plus a soft vinyl (a low-coast athletic mouth guard) splint (SS). The evaluation was peformed at 3, 6 and 12 months. They reported that all the patients showed improvement over time, and traditional splint therapy offered no benefit over the SS splint therapy. Neither splint therapy provided a greater benefit than did self-care treatment without splint therapy.

The UT included jaw relaxation, reduction of parafunction, thermal pack, NSAIDs, passive opening stretches and suggestions about stress reduction (Truelove E *et al.*, 2006). Wassel *et al.* evaluated TMD outcomes in general dental practice one year after treatment with stabilizing splints (SS) or non-occluding control splint (CS). They reported that after one year, good response to TMD treatment in general practice was maintained, but various subjects still reported clicking TMJs. It was observed that after initial treatment, only six subjects according to predefined criteria needed occlusal adjustment. The criteria maintained that on splint removal, the subject experienced the return of pain with the evidence of occlusal interference, an awareness of an uncomfortable occlusion or both (Wassel RW *et al.*, 2006). Conti *et al.* compared the efficacy of bilateral balanced and canine guidance (occlusal) splints in the treatment of TMJ pain in subjects who experienced joint clicking with a nonoccluding splint in a double-blind, controlled randomized clinical trial. They reported that the type of lateral guidance did not influence the subjects' improvement. All subjects showed general improvement on the VAS, though subjects in the occlusal splint groups displayed better results than did subjects in the nonoccluding splint group (Conti PC et al., 2006).

Alencar and Becker compared the effectiveness of different occlusal splints (hard, soft or non-occluding occlusal splint) associated with counselling and self-care in the management of signs and symptoms of myofascial pain. They reported that all patients improved over time and all splints offered the benefit (Alencar F, Jr. & Becker A, 2009). Splint therapies and self-care are symptomatic therapies, not causal therapies. Therfore, it needs to be confirmed that no recurrence occurs on splint removal as described by Wassel et al (Wassel RW et al., 2006).

3. OUTCOME OF OCCLUSAL TREATMENT

Mejersjö and Carlsson reported subjective and objective findings on examination of a group of patients 7 years after evaluation and treatment for TMJ pain-dysfunction symptoms. They described that treatments given to 154 patients with TMD were; 100%: counseling; 75%: occlusal adjustment; 74%: therapeutic exercises; 58%: splint; 30%: physical therapy; 18%: prosthetic treatment; 10%: injection; 8%: increased vertical dimension of occlusion (temporary); 7%: systemic (pharmacotherapy); and 1%: orthodontic treatment. The results of the 7-year examination were compared with the records made prior to treatment. There was a significant reduction in both the reported symptoms and clinical signs of dysfunction at 7 years. Although less severe than at initial examination, clicking of the TMJ and slight muscle tenderness to palpation were the most common clinical findings at 7 years. Eighty-four percent of patients reported that the treatment received resulted in the reduction of symptoms. During the 7-year period, 80% of patients showed few or no symptoms. Recurrent symptoms of some significance were found in less than 20% of patients, and 14% returned for further treatment during the 7-year period. It can be concluded that most patients with TMJ pain-dysfunction reported minimal recurrent symptoms 7 years after conservative treatment procedures. This indicates that a favorable prognosis may be considered for TMJ pain dysfunction. This favorable prognosis should be emphasized to patients prior to treatment, as optimistic counseling has been shown to have a favorable effect on patient's response to treatment (Mejersjö C & Carlsson GE, 1983). The data indicate that clinical signs of TMJ clicking or muscle pain were not resolved and the treatment included occlusal adjustment, which was not conservative treatment. Torii and Chiwata performed a pilot study of occlusal adjustment using the bite plate-induced occlusal position as a reference position for TMDs (Torii K & Chiwata I, 2010). Their treatment method was described in Chapter 7. The distribution of dysfunction indices before occlusal adjustment is shown in Fig. **1**.

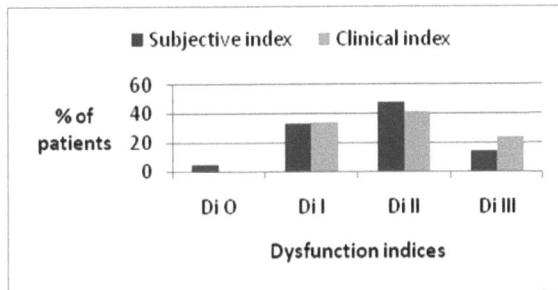

Figure 1: Dysfunction indices at first examination.

Distribution of dysfunction indices before occlusal adjustment: Di O: no TMD; Di I: mild TMD; Di II: moderate TMD; Di III: severe TMD.

The distribution of dysfunction indices after occlusal adjustment is shown in Fig. **2**.

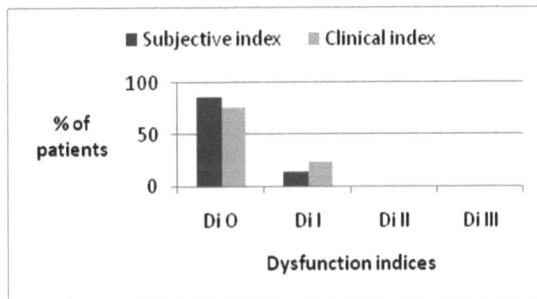

Figure 2: Dysfunction indices at 1-year evaluation.

Distribution of dysfunction indices after occlusal adjustment: Di O: no TMD; Di I: mild TMD; Di II: moderate TMD; Di III: severe TMD.

None of the patients required an anterior bite plate during their one-year follow-up period after the completion of the occlusal adjustment. The number of visits varied between 2 and 34, with a mean of 11.0±6.0 visits. The treatment period ranged between 0.2 and 7.0 months, with a mean of 2.8±2.1 months. The bite plate wearing period ranged from 1 to 21 days, with a mean of 9.6±6.7 days. Around 13 sessions of occlusal adjustment were performed, with a mean of 4.7±3.5 sessions. The subjective index (SDI) had a median value of 9, ranging between 7 and 17 at the time of first examination, and 1 after the one-year follow-up. The change was statistically significant (p<0.01). The clinical dysfunction index (CDI) decreased from a median value of 9 before treatment to 1 after treatment. This change was also significant (p<0.01). Changes in the frequencies of headaches are shown in Fig. **3**. The frequency significantly lowered after occlusal adjustment. Thirteen patients reported headache symptoms.

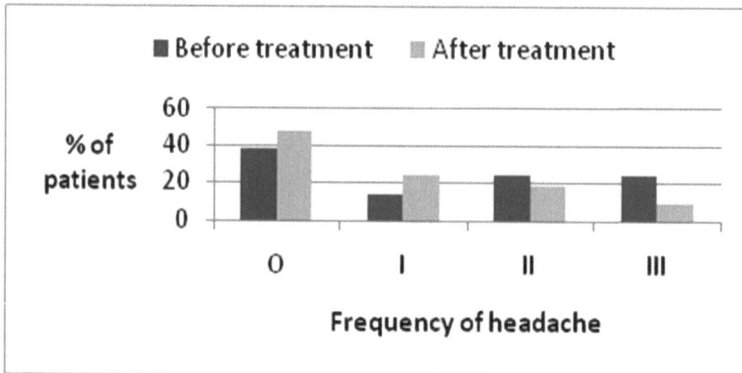

Figure 3: Headache frequency before and after treatment.

Five of changes in headache frequency before and after occlusal adjustment: O: almost never; I: 1 to 2 times a month; II: 1 to 2 times a week; III: every day. These patients did not experience any further headache after treatment. The scores of 8 of the 13 patients with headache symptoms improved by 1 or 2 score categories. The distribution of graded chronic pain on Axis II of RDC/TMD was as follows: grade 0, 3 patients (14%); grade 1, 12 patients (57%); and grade 2, 6 patients (29%) before treatment. After treatment, all patients had a grade 0. The changes in the mean difference between the HOP and BPOP before and after occlusal adjustment are shown in Fig. **4**. The changes in the mean difference on the x-axis (mediolateral) and y-axis (anteroposterior) were significant ($p<0.05$), whereas the change on the z-axis (superoinferior) was not significant ($p>0.1$). The changes in the statistical difference between the HOP and BPOP after treatment were significant (Table **1**).

Table 1: Changes in the statistical difference between the HOP and BPOP before and after treatment

Before occlusal adjustment	After Occlusal Adjustment	
	No difference	Difference
Difference	20	0
No difference	1	0

McNemar's test: $x^2_{cal} = 18.05 > x^2_1 (0.001) = 10.83$, Significant.

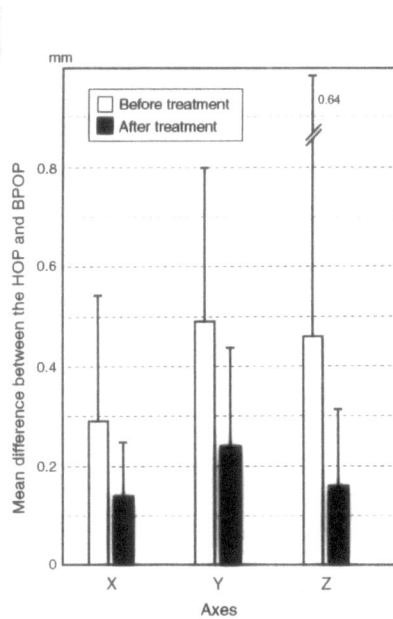

Figure 4: Mean HOP-BPOP difference before and after treatment.

Changes in the mean difference between the habitual occlusal position (HOP) and the bite plate-induced occlusal position (BPOP) before and after occlusal adjustment. X: mediolateral; Y: anteroposterior and Z: superoinferior.

Regarding subtypes of TMD, the mean number of visits were 12.8±6.9 visits for myofascial pain, 10.3±4.9 visits for disc displacement and 13.9±8.1 visits for arthritis. The mean lengths of the treatment periods were 3.5±1.2 months for myofascial pain, 1.9±1.5 months for disc disc displacement and 3.6±2.1 months for arthritis. The mean number of occlusal adjustments were 6.8 times for myofacial pain, 4.0±3.1 times for disc displacement and 4.5±0.7 times for arthritis. No significant difference in the mean number of visits, mean lengths of the treatment period, or the mean number of occlusal adjustments was observed among the three TMD subtypes when the differences were analyzed using t-tests. The outcomes of the occlusal adjustments for TMD subtypes are shown in Table **2**.

Table 2: Changes in Helkimo Clinical Dysfunction Index at first examination and after a 1-year follow-up examination for each TMD subtype.

CDI	Myofascial Pain		Disc Displacement		Arthritis	
	1st Exam	1 y	1st Exam	1 y	1st Exam	1 y
Di O	0%	80%	0%	86%	0%	0%
Di I	0%	20%	36%	14%	0%	100%
Di II	40%	0%	43%	0%	50%	0%
Di III	20%	0%	21%	0%	50%	0%

CDI: Helkimo Clinical Index; 1st Exam.: first examination; 1 y: 1-year follow-up examination; Di O: no TMD; Di I: mild TMD; Di II: moderate TMD; Di III: severe TMD.

The outcomes of occlusal equilibration with prosthesis are shown in Table **3**.

Table 3: Outcome of occlusal equilibration in the muscular contact position with prosthesis.

No.	Age	Gender	Complaints	Diagnosis	Period	Outcome	Follow-up Period	
1	41	F	Left TMJ Pain	Disc NR	16 months	resolved	22 years	No recur.
2	50	M	Left TMJ Pain	Disc NR	4 months	resolved	17 years.	No recur.
3	61	M	Right TMJ Pain	Disc NR	12 months	resolved	5 years	No recur.
4	75	F	Both TMJ Pain	Disc NR	5 months	resolved	10 months	No recur.
5	54	M	Right TMJ Pain	Disc NR	5 months	resolved	2 months	No recur.
6	44	F	Left TMJ Pain	Disc NR	4 years	resolved	23 years	No recur.
7	50	F	Right TMJ Pain	Disc NR	2 months	resolved	1 year	No recur.
8	38	F	Right TMJ Pain	Disc NR	5 months	resolved	25 years	No recur.
9	76	M	Right TMJ Pain	Disc NR	2 months	resolved	6 months	No recur.
10	72	F	Right TMJ Pain	Disc NR	2 months	resolved	1.5 years	No recur.

No.: Patient number; Period: treatment period; Disc NR: Disc displacement without reduction; No recur.: No recurrence; F: Female; M: Male.

Patient No. 4 had severe symptoms of difficulty in walking, rotating the neck and mouth opening. She visited two orthopedic clinics, and thereafter visited a general hospital. She then received an injection into the lumbar, but the injection failed to improve her severe symptoms and she visited for follow-up the same day. She complained of pain in the left TMJ. An anterior flat bite plate was fabricated directly in her mouth, and she worn it. She was asked to tap her teeth against it, while she was received laser therapy on the left TMJ for 20 minutes. The amount of month opening changed from 25 mm to 42 mm after the therapies. When her pain subsided, the wedge shaped spaces on both molar region emerged in the muscular contact position (that is BPOP) which were filled with teeth restorations. Among patients in Table **3**, only patient No. 9 was treated with upper complete denture and lower partial denture and rest of the patients were treated with fixed prosthesis. Table **4** shows the outcome of occlusal adjustment in the BPOP for patients with aural symptoms related to TMD.

Table 4: Treatment outcome of TMD patients with aural symptoms

No.	Age	Gender	Complaints	Diagnosis	Period	Outcome	Follow-up period
1	16	M	Limited Opening Tinnitus (R), Headache	Disc R (R)	2 months	resolved	5 years No recurrence
2	20	F	Limited opening Tinnitus (R)	Disc R (B) Myofascial	5 months	resolved	3 years No recurrence
3	22	F	Limited opening Headache, Tinnitus (L), Myofascial	Disc R (L)	5 months	resolved	3 years No recurrence
4	28	F	Limited opening Tinnitus (L), fullness	Myofascial (L)	3 months	resolved	5 years No recurrence
5	35	F	Facial pain Headache, tinnitus (L)	Myofascial (L)	2 months	resolved	3 years No recurrence
6	37	F	Limited opening Tinnitus (L), headache	Disc R (L)	3 months	resolved	10 years No recurrence
7	42	F	Facial pain Tinnitus (L), vertigo	Myofascial (L)	2 months	resolved	5 years No recurrence
8	47	F	Limited opening Tinnitus (L)	Disc R (L)	5 months	resolved	2 years No recurrence
9	73	F	TMJ pain Vertigo (R), tinnitus (R)	Arthralgia (R)	5 months	resolved	7 years No recurrence

No.: Patient number; Period: Treatment period; Disc R: Disc displacement with reduction; Myofascial: Myofascial pain; M: Male; F: Female; (R), (L) and (B): Mainly affected side on the (R): right; (L): left; (B): both side.

All the patients in Table **4** were treated only with occlusal adjustment in the muscular contact position. In evaluating the outcome of treatment, it is important to confirm that every clinical symptom and sign of TMD (pain and limitations in all mandibular movements, clicking of TMJ, deviation in opening mouth, and tenderness of masticatory muscles and TMJ to palpation) is completely disappeared.

SUMMARY

It is a serious problem that conservative therapies could not resolve severe TMD symptoms. We should make greater effort to relieve the patients suffering from severe TMD symptoms.

REFERENCES

Alencar F, Jr. & Becker A (2009). Evaluation of different occlusal splints and counseling in the management of myofascial pain dysfunction. *J Oral Rehabil* 2009;36:79-85.

De Boever JA, Van Den Berghe L, De Boever AL, Keersmaekers K (1999). Comparison of clinical profiles and treatment outcomes of an elderly and a younger temporomandibular patient group. *J Prosthet Dent* 1999;81:312-317.

Conti PC, dos Santos CN, Kogawa EM, de Castro Ferreira Conti AC, de Araujo C dos RP (2006). The treatment of painful temporomandibular joint clicking with oral splints: a randomized clinical trial. *J Am Dent Assoc* 2006;137:1108-1114.

Ekberg E, Vallon D, Nlner M (2003). The efficacy of appliance therapy in patients with temporomandibular disorders of mainly myogenous origin. A randomized, controlled, short-term trial. *J Orofac Pain* 2003;17:133139.

Greene CS & Laskin DM (1983). Long-term evaluation of treatment for myofascial pain-dysfunction syndrome: a comparative analysis. *J Am Dent Assoc* 1983;107:235-238.

Mejersjö C & Carlsson GE (1983). Long-term results of treatment for temporomandibular joint-pain dysfunction. *J Prosthet Dent* 1983;49:807-815.

Schmitter M, Zahran M, Duc JM, Henschel V, Rammelsberg P (2005). Conservative therapy in patients with anterior disc displacement without reduction using 2 common splints: a randomized clinical trial. *L Oral Maxillofac Surg* 2005;63:1295-1303.

Torii K & Chiawata I (2010). Occlusal adjustment using the bite plate-induced occlusal position as a reference position for temporomandibular disorders: a pilot study. *Head & Face Medicine* 2010, 6:5. Available from: http://www.head-face-med.com/content/6/1/5

Truelove E, Huggins KH, Mancl L, Dworkin SF (2006). The efficacy of traditional, low cost and nonsplint therapies for temporomandibular disorder: a randomized controlled trial. *J Am Dent Assoc* 2006;137:1099-1107.

Wassell RW, Adams N, Kelly PJ (2006). The treatment of tempromandibular disorders with stabilizing splints in general dental practice: one-year follow-up. *J Am Dent Assoc* 2006;137:1089-1099.

Index

A

Acupuncture treatment   103

ADR   143-4, 168-70

Adrenocorticotropin   157

Afferent impulses   62-3, 67

Analyzing occlusal adjustment   45

Analyzing rods   129-30, 139

Angiotensin-converting enzyme (ACE)   181

Anterior mandibular movement   105

Anterior positioning splint   103

Anterior repositioning splint   146

Anterior-superior position   35

Anterior temporal   45

Anterior temporal muscles   21, 45

Anterior temporalis muscles   107

Antero-posterior   56-8

Anterolateral movement   105

Antigravity muscles   61, 150

Arrow point contact position   83

Arthrogenous craniomandibular pain   113

Arthrogenous pain   113

Arthropathic TMJ   167-8

Articulare   76-7

Articulator techniques   66, 68

Artificial occlusal discrepancy   158

Asymmetric slides   42

B

Balancing interferences   22

Balancing-side interferences   46, 68

O

P

www.ingramcontent.com/pod-product-compliance
Lightning Source LLC
Chambersburg PA
CBHW041727210326
41598CB00008B/801

* 9 7 8 1 6 0 8 0 5 7 8 4 9 *